# Praise for *Pet Goats & Pap Smears*

"Dr. Wible changes our profession's national conversation from misery to joy, from despair to hope as she describes building her dream clinic. This book has challenges and lessons for all."
~ L. Gordon Moore, M.D., president of Ideal Medical Practices

"I laughed and cried while reading these stories in between patients."
~ Adolfo E. Teran, M.D., medical director of Orange Doc Family Medicine

"Dr. Wible's book is addictive. Rarely does one get to see the human heart and soul expressed so beautifully in one's job. A must-read for all medical students, physicians, and patients."
~ Mark J. McGinley, M.D., medical director of Wyoming Medical Center ICU

"My eight-year-old son—barely a reader and hardly a writer—asks, 'What are you reading?' I reply, 'Pamela Wible's book.' He exclaims, 'Wow, she wrote a book?' Later, he announces, 'I'm going to write my life story.' Not only has Dr. Wible started a movement to counter quick-fix, impersonal, and institutionalized medicine, but she has also inspired me to open my own clinic and my son to write his memoir!"
~ Angela Heithaus, M.D., self-employed in Seattle

"Not your usual, boring medical book. Freaky, a little weird, and very educational."
~ Julian Safar, high school student in Oregon

"A joyful read that touches the soul, *Pet Goats & Pap Smears* made me laugh, smile, and hold my heart. Dr. Wible is a true healer."
~ Anandhi Mandi, M.D., founder of Dr. Mandi's Integrative Pediatrics

"Hallelujah! A book that celebrates the honored tradition of the doctor-patient relationship. Dr. Pamela Wible shares intimate moments with patients that will make you smile and feel reassured that warm, caring, and passionate doctors still exist."
~ Amy Solomon, M.D., founder of Balance Health of Ben Lomond

"Dr. Pamela Wible is a visionary and a storyteller. *Pet Goats & Pap Smears* is the perfect combination of quirky, heartwarming, and hilarious."
~ Leila Ali-Akbarian, M.D., M.P.H., assistant professor, University of Arizona Department of Family Medicine

"Here's an alternative to churn-and-burn primary care teams: jump off the hamster wheel and allow patients to create the clinic of their dreams."
~ Kristin L. Oaks, D.O., founder of an ideal medical clinic in Ohio

"I was ready to quit medicine for a job as a Walmart greeter. *Pet Goats & Pap Smears* has rekindled my spirit and salvaged my career. This how-to-be-a-happy-healer handbook is the perfect gift for every doctor—and patient. Give a copy to your family doc! The life you save may save you."
~ Tricia Williams, M.D., planning her practice in Pennsylvania

"I met Pamela at a conference she offered—at *no* cost to physicians—where she encouraged us to answer one question: 'What is ideal health care?' This question changed my life. I just resigned from my job to open my ideal clinic! I'm eternally grateful for Dr. Wible and her book. She helped me figure out *how* to bring joy back to my daily medical practice. I, in turn, vow to do whatever I can to help other physicians practice medicine with the love and joy she so selflessly shared with me. Pamela also found me a husband (or at least a good romance)!"
~ Sheila Kilbane, M.D., opening her ideal clinic in Charlotte, North Carolina

"*Pet Goats & Pap Smears* takes you on a journey of the heart and brings love and laughter to a health system that is sorely lacking both. Pamela Wible's inspiration will surely change the face of modern medicine. Imagine creating your ideal clinic! Why not? Pamela has given me the impetus to create my dream clinic in Albuquerque. Thank you Pamela!"
~ Sunil Pai, M.D., founder of Sanjevani Integrative Medicine Health & Lifestyle Center

"Whether it's a speculum or a pet goat, one size does not fit all. Excellent health care meets patients where they are. May Pamela Wible continue to inspire us all!"
~ Myria Emeny, M.D., founder of Doc Myria's Family Practice

"A tantalizing peek behind the primary-care curtain where all barriers between doctor and patient have come down."
~ Lynn Ho, M.D., enjoying her ideal practice in Rhode Island

"Pamela Wible is one of the most inspiring, creative, and courageous physicians in America today. Her voice speaks to what is possible in the transformation of health care in the United States. *Pet Goats & Pap Smears* invites us to open our hearts and to reconnect with ourselves and the visions that led us to become healers in the first place. Dr. Wible shows us such a simple solution to the health care crisis: it's called caring for people."
~ Maxine Barish-Wreden, M.D., medical director of Sutter Center for
Integrative Holistic Medicine

"Here's a book for doctors contemplating early retirement in the prime of their careers. *Pet Goats & Pap Smears* celebrates the sustainable, solo primary care practices that are popping up all over the country. Don't retire. Join us! It *is* possible to live, laugh, and love medicine again."

~ Lisa Quillin, M.D., founder of Quillin Family Medicine

"Want to change the world? Try peace, love, and pet goats."

~ Jordan Dearon Wells, student at McNeese State University

"In this joyous and uplifting book, Dr. Wible captures the essence of the patient-physician relationship. This is how many physicians visualized themselves practicing medicine, but only a few hold on to the dream. A great read for everyone—and a must-read for every medical student."

~ Alok Kalia, M.D., clinical professor of pediatrics, University of Texas Medical Branch-Galveston

"Thank you, Pamela, for reaffirming that I can LOVE practicing medicine. I can't wait to share these stories with my classmates."

~ Michael Latteri, medical student at Oregon Health & Science University

"What a joy! What an inspiration! Every one of our family medicine residents should take a heaping dose of *Pet Goats & Pap Smears*. This is good medicine for all that ails health care in the United States—and it's just what the doctor ordered for happy healers everywhere!"

~ Dónal Kevin Gordon, M.D., program director of Cedar Rapids Family Medicine Residency

"Awesome. Hysterical. This book is #MedicalSwag."

~ Haley Krouse, premedical student in Pennsylvania

"In today's broken health care system, doctors have lost sight of what is most important: serving patients. Dr. Wible's solution is powerful in its simplicity: rediscover the sacred doctor-patient relationship. I'm so inspired by her that I opened my own ideal clinic."

~ Orestes Gutierrez, D.O., assistant professor of family medicine, Western University of Health Science

"Pamela Wible is leading the charge against impersonal health care with a superb alternative: design your dream clinic. These delightful tales document exactly why she is wildly successful and how the rest of us can join her pioneering revolution for personalized and sane health care."

~ Sara Gottfried, M.D., author of *The Hormone Cure*

"A breath of fresh air! In a health care system overtaken by protocols and check-lists, Dr. Wible articulates the true art of medicine: it's about cultivating relation-ships with patients. Physicians and medical students, take off your white coats and come down off that pedestal, for this is required reading!"

~ Jeffrey Gladd, M.D., founder of GladdMD Integrative Medicine

"I learned more in a few pages of this book than I did in my high school health class."

~ Phebe Udo, student at University of Oregon

"I laughed, I cried, I dreamt. I always wanted to open a solo practice, but had many fears. Now I realize that all I need is the enthusiasm and patient-centered approach that Dr. Wible models in her vignettes. This book will reinvigorate readers who have let medicine beat them down. You *can* practice medicine the way you have always dreamed!"

~ Maya Porrino, M.D., graduate of the Arizona Center for Integrative Medicine

"*Pet Goats & Pap Smears* is touching, funny, sad, and inspirational. As a former miserable doctor who has found happiness in a practice similar to Pamela's, I can attest to the drastic need for THIS kind of health care reform—for both patients and doctors. Pamela Wible is a visionary who can help save us from ourselves. My prescription: read her book."

~ Lonna Larsh, M.D., founder of Holistic Family Doctor

"Pamela Wible lovingly challenges physicians to offer the kind of medicine that most of us dreamed about when we entered medical school. She is not calling for more martyrs—she is calling for patients and physicians to experience more fun, joy, and happiness. Very, very, wholeheartedly inspiring."

~ Lissa Lubinski, M.D., rural full-spectrum family physician and mother

"Dr. Wible is resuscitating our nearly dead medical profession with humor, love, and common sense!"

~ Jolaine Beal, M.D., M.P.H., dreaming of her ideal clinic in Berkeley

"An awesome way to learn about all the random things you want to know."

~ Jamie Satterwhite, high school student in Oregon

"Wonderful stories! A front-row seat to the human drama through the eyes, ears, and heart of a healer and revolutionary—silly, profound, and a balm to the wounded soul of modern health care."

~ John Glick, M.D., director of Gesundheit Institute Global Outreach

"A book of funny, sad, and inspiring stories of hope and encouragement, *Pet Goats & Pap Smears* stirs the emotions and provides optimism in a malfunctioning medical system. Why don't doctors go into solo practice? With huge student loans and no salary guarantee, a corporate sellout of our souls is enticing. Thank you, Pamela, for bringing us back to the humanity of practicing medicine!"
~ Elaine Chu, M.D., author of *What It Takes To Be Healthy*


"Pamela's writing has given me even more motivation and inspiration to become the excellent, caring doctor I've always wanted to be."
~ Rachel Bigley, premedical student at University of California, Berkeley


"*Pet Goats & Pap Smears* provides a genuine alternative vision for the practice and business of medicine. Dr. Wible's view will resonate with every patient who has ever been frustrated by the self-serving side of American medicine. The wonderful two years I practiced with Dr. Wible confirm firsthand that she also has the skills to impress a traditional family physician like me."
~ Michael R. Boyd, M.D., former president of Olympia Family Medicine


"In an effort to deliver evidence-based, patient-centered, quality medical care, today's average doc has forgotten to pay attention to the real evidence: the patient. Finally, it is Pamela Wible who is putting a stop to this health-care-delivery-system insanity."
~ Aylin Ozdemir, M.D., F.A.A.P., founder of Dr. O Integrative Medical Centers, Jacksonville, Florida


"Dr. Wible's groundbreaking book digs into the truth-and-dare of her bold, grass-roots movement to restore the patient-physician relationship. Honest, moving, and inspirational, *Pet Goats & Pap Smears* is a must-read for anyone who has ever given or received health care!"
~ Jennifer Griffin, M.D., founder of Integrative Family Medicine


"Pamela Wible is a rare find—a physician who has managed to hold on to her sense of humor, compassion, and feisty passion for healing. In *Pet Goats & Pap Smears* she reminds us of the potential for beauty and creativity in the physician-patient relationship."
~ Lara Knudsen, M.D., M.P.H., author of *Reproductive Rights in a Global Context*


"Dr. Wible brings to life a real sampling of doctor-patient relationships that can only develop in small, caring practice settings."
~ Ron Edwards, M.D., founder of Family Health Topeka in Kansas

"An inspiration! *Pet Goats & Pap Smears* helped me remember why I became a doctor in the first place. Pamela's guidance has shown me the way out of corporate medicine to a place where I can truly take care of patients—my own practice."

~ Heather Shelton, M.D., founder of Green Island Health in Fort Worth, Texas

"Pamela Wible, a conventionally trained family physician, uses her amazing out-of-the-box thinking to make her dream of an ideal medical clinic a reality. *Pet Goats & Pap Smears* takes us along on her pilgrimage to the heart of the patient-physician relationship. These stories made me laugh, cry, and question the way we teach and practice medicine."

~ Patricia Lebensohn, M.D., professor of clinical family and community medicine, University of Arizona

"An interesting, upbeat, and seriously fun book about practicing medicine. *Pet Goats & Pap Smears* is the doctor's guide to achieving peace of mind through a good sense of humor."

~ Rosalia Leite Evans, M.D., M.P.H., founder of Palm Beach Hello Health

"Dr. Wible is ingenious, innovative, and inspiring. *Pet Goats & Pap Smears* proves that happy doctors can heal the health care system."

~ Evan H. Hirsch, M.D., medical director of Providence Integrative Cancer Care

"In 2005, I was on sabbatical in Italy when I began plotting my own practice. Pamela was one of the few doctors who encouraged me to open my practice out of my home. I didn't know her—except in virtual reality, through a group of doctors online—but her stories revealed the raw truth and humanity of caring for patients. Now, after building a successful home-based practice, I help others open their ideal clinics. May her stories also inspire you to make your own dream come true."

~ Sharon McCoy George, M.D., associate clinical professor of medicine, University of California-Irvine

"I love *Pet Goats & Pap Smears*! I learned a ton!"

~ Chloe Safar, eighth-grade student in Oregon

"Pamela's book is not about entertaining, fictional characters, but real people whose happiness, pain, humor, and wisdom leap off the pages to inspire us all—doctors and patients. Though amusing and light in places, this book is also thought provoking and, indeed, revolutionary. You can't just read this book. You must chew it and digest it and let it become part of you."

~ Jina Shah, M.D., M.P.H., clinical instructor of family and community medicine, University of California, San Francisco

"Dr. Wible is one of the most influential writers of our time."

~ Cyrus Peikari, M.D., author of *Internal Medicine Board Review*

# Pet Goats &
# Pap Smears™

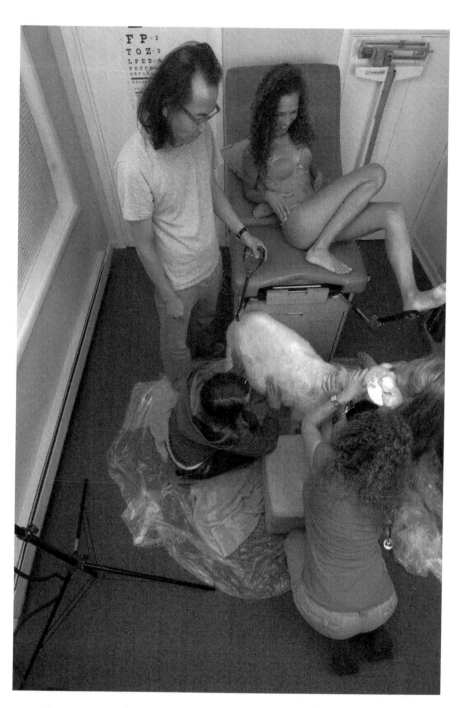

If you're wondering if the goat was photoshopped—she wasn't.

# Pet Goats & Pap Smears™

## 101 Medical Adventures to Open Your Heart & Mind

Pamela Wible, M.D.

with illustrations by
Kiki Metzler

Pamela Wible, M.D., Publishing
Oregon

www.petgoatsandpapsmears.com

Library of Congress Control Number: 2012914951

ISBN: 978-0-9857103-0-9

Illustrations: Kiki Metzler
Editing: Betsy Robinson, Bo Adan
Design and Production: Kassy Daggett


PHOTO CREDITS:
Front Cover ~ Wind Home
Back Cover ~ Digital Latte
Pages x, 64, 239, 241 ~ Wind Home
Page 11 ~ Jim Young, Page 34 ~ Bob Specht
Pages 49, 131, 132, 236 ~ Judith Wible
Page 99 ~ Anil Namboodiripad, Page 157 ~ Ted Krouse
Page 161 ~ Unknown, Pages 206, 209 ~ Pamela Wible
Page 217 ~ Surya Narayana, Page 240 ~ Laura Apgar

*Dedicated to all premedical and medical students*
*and to every child who has ever dreamed of being a doctor.*

# Table of Contents

## I. On Service

## II. On Joy

## III. On Creativity

## IV. On Compassion

## V. On Teaching

## VI. On Intuition

## VII. On Love

## VIII. On Death

# TABLE OF CONTENTS

# Foreword

Pamela Wible . . . YES!

I started reading Pamela's new book, hoping, with my schedule, to finish it in two weeks. As soon as I began reading the book, I couldn't put it down. For the first time in forty-five years, I have found a physician who has explored the practice of medicine as I have. Thank you, Pamela, for being a living example of possibility.

In 2008, Pamela and I met over the subject of designing health care delivery systems. In 2009, we invited her to present at our *Thinking Outside the Box* conference. We wanted people at our event who are hungering for a fun, enchanting way to practice medicine, and Pamela is this kind of person.

*Pet Goats & Pap Smears* presents stories of sweetness in the practice of medicine. Pamela's stories are so delicious, you want to be a doctor. I will now recommend this book to all students of health care at any level. Pamela says relax, love your patients, experience friendship and play, listen with every cell of your body, be vulnerable and interested, and see the clear richness of life all along the way. Yes! I can't wait until our hospital is built, so Pamela can play doctor with us.

Please, reader, if you create your ideal medical practice, make it like this. The practice of medicine is one of love's dances. Dr. Wible lays it out here, the gold mine (mind) of medicine. Be the doctor you always dreamed of being. Practice medicine exactly as you choose. You decide. This book is a decide guide. Dive in! Whee!

In Peace,
Patch Adams, M.D.

# Introduction

Hi, I'm Pamela.

I'm a family physician born into a family of physicians. Mom is a psychiatrist. Dad is an addiction specialist and pathologist at the hospital morgue. I spent my childhood playing in hospital hallways and stairwells. I loved the morgue. Dad made it fun. He talked to the dead people in the coolers, so I did too. From the morgue, we made our rounds to the city jail, drug addiction clinic, and the psychiatric hospital. Introduced as a doctor-in-training, I was set loose on inmates, heroin addicts, and schizophrenics while most girls my age were playing with Barbies.

My dream was to be an amazing doctor—like my mom and dad, only better. My parents warned me not to pursue medicine. They said government regulation and bureaucracy were killing the old-fashioned family doctor. But there was no way to stop me. I had already made up my mind.

Family doctors are the kind of doctors who do everything. I planned to deliver babies and help people die, plus treat criminals and people on drugs and people nobody else could help. Maybe I'd be a medical superhero and save an entire city. I'd go on midnight house calls by flying from town to town in my white cape, pockets overflowing with get-well stickers and cherry-flavored tongue depressors. Like most kids, I believed that being a superhero was a practical career choice. So I ignored my parents' warnings and went to medical school and then graduated from residency in family and community medicine.

My first job was at a big clinic in Oregon. I didn't feel heroic. I felt like a factory worker pushing pills into patients as they flew past me on a conveyor belt. I tried other jobs, but they were all the same—assembly-line medicine. Doctoring was dumbed down to a numbers game with cookbook protocols and computerized flowsheets. Patients were often excluded from care if they had no insurance or if they took too long to express themselves. Or if they were shy or different or addicted to heroin or in jail. Or if they were not easy, simple, healthy middle-aged people with good insurance and minor health problems.

Eventually I left all those jobs to pursue my dream.

This book shows how, with persistence, I came to live my dream. I hope my story inspires you to live your dream even when people tell you it's not possible. Revolutionary ideas start as dreams. If nobody understands your dream, it's okay. *You* are the visionary.


## A Dream Clinic Is Born

After ten years on the treadmill, I was tired of being rude to people and neglecting myself—all in the name of health care. I hated interrupting patients to say, "Sorry, we're out of time," when I wanted to ask, "How can I help you?" So I dropped out of medicine and imagined returning to my college waitressing job just so I could be nice to people again. At least when I was a waitress, people appreciated me. And they left tips.

When I gave up doctoring, life seemed meaningless. I fell into a depression and didn't get out of bed for six weeks.

Then—in a dream—came an epiphany: patients could create their own clinics! In my dream, I saw grandmothers and grandchildren, teachers and teenagers, farmers and firefighters—entire communities—coming together to build ideal clinics and hospitals.

Energized, I jumped out of bed. Feeling invincible, I phoned the newspaper and told the editor that I'd be opening an ideal clinic created entirely by our community. Then I called a series of town hall meetings and invited citizens to design the clinic of their dreams. I collected 100 pages of testimony, adopted ninety percent of the feedback, and opened our clinic one month later! In 2005, the people of Eugene, Oregon, had created the first community-designed ideal clinic in America.

Now reporters fly here from all over the country to study our clinic. Hundreds of ideal clinics have opened nationwide. Communities have even used our model to design ideal hospitals. I now know that just by living my dream, I can inspire others to live their dreams too.

# Why Pet Goats? Why Pap Smears?

## Why Pet Goats?

As I led town halls across America, pet goats were an unexpected theme in citizen testimony. And to my surprise, pet goats keep popping up in my life. The healing potential of animals is underutilized in medicine. Who knows? Maybe this year I'll find that special goat for our clinic, or I'll offer Pap smears at a petting zoo, if that's what my patients want. While editing this paragraph, I'm introduced to a lady who has a mobile petting zoo—with fifteen goats! No kidding.

## Why Pap Smears?

A Pap smear is a screening test for cervical cancer, in which a smear of cervical cells is taken from inside a woman's vagina. The cervix is the doorway to the womb, the birthplace of all humanity. When I'm in between my patients' thighs looking deep inside the places where nobody has looked before, patients often tell me things that they've never shared with anybody. This sacred relationship between a doctor and patient is the foundation of health care.

I work in a gold mine of human drama and comedy. For twenty years, patients have been telling me their stories. I can no longer contain them; now, I release their stories to the world. Here, I give voice to the voiceless and credibility to incredible lives. I've written about patients in previous books, yet the more I write, the more patients plead, "Have I made it into your next book?" So I keep writing.

Inside me live the stories of dead patients too. I heard their last words. Now—through my words—patients live again.

*Pet Goats & Pap Smears* is more than a collection of stories. It's a book of 101 medical adventures that have been retrieved from the deepest places inside people I have cared for. Sometimes, I'm so deep inside patients that I believe I have touched their souls. I know they have touched mine.

## Why This Book Now?

Health care can never be mandated. Most people suffer ill health from poor lifestyle choices. Legislation can support healthy behavior, but laws can't force people to care about themselves—or anyone else. Compassion comes from the heart, not the pen. Caring is a personal choice born from an awakening of the heart and soul.

Health care can never be mandated from the top down, because what Americans really want comes from the inside out and the bottom up.

Doctors are the heart of health care. But doctors are discouraged. Overwhelmed and underappreciated, most doctors have considered quitting medicine. Malpractice fears have turned the physician-patient relationship from sacred to scared. In these pages, you'll peek inside the hearts and souls of America's doctors. Here is where health care reform begins. I offer this book to help heal our wounded healers.

Happy doctors don't retire early. Happy doctors don't abandon direct patient care for administrative positions in pharmaceutical or insurance companies. And they don't leave medicine for waitressing. I've learned that it *is* financially viable to practice medicine in alignment with one's highest values and the values of one's community.

America needs happy doctors.

*Pet Goats & Pap Smears* goes where other books have never been. These pages delve deep inside real people to uncover the moral and political conflicts of our day. Explore prostitution, medical marijuana, animal rights, physician-assisted suicide, and capital punishment from inside the bodies of my patients.

It's not my job to judge patients. I invite you to decide whether our laws and behaviors with one another are ethical and just.

May you enjoy the journey.

# Who Should Read This Book?

## Premedical & Medical Students

This book offers what medical school doesn't.

Medical training teaches technical skills, but not the art of medicine. Doctors are taught to order blood tests and CAT scans, to diagnose and drug, to perform surgery. But we have no courses on how to serve patients with joy. We have no textbooks on love and compassion. We aren't tested on creativity. Intuition is rarely recognized as a diagnostic tool. And all too often, we view death as our own failure. Trained to detach emotionally and spiritually from patients, medical students eventually lose connection with the meaning of life and the mystery of death.

While speaking to an undergraduate medical humanities class, I was shocked to discover that students today are still taught "professional distance." The professor warned me that his class was unlikely to be participatory, but when I described our community clinic, students burst forth with questions: "It's okay to let patients call you *Pamela*? You pray with patients? Is it legal to hug them?" Most patients call me Pamela. I eat, pray, and laugh with them. Sometimes, I cry with them. And it's still legal to hug.

That evening I spoke to premedical students. Afterward, a group congregated around me. They said, "We've never met a solo doctor. Or a happy doctor." One woman shared, "We don't have any mentors. Can we visit your office and shadow you?"

"Of course! Come visit anytime and spend an afternoon seeing patients with me."

Here, I offer myself as a mentor to all the students who will never have the opportunity to hang out with me at our community clinic. I have written this book for you.

## Doctors & Patients

To my colleagues who are cynical and suffering, may these stories reignite your passion for medicine. Keep this book on your desk and in the exam room as a reference. Put the e-book in your white-coat pocket. *Pet Goats & Pap Smears* may be the best medicine for you and your patients. Sharing a story can be more potent than writing a prescription.

Patients, enjoy a story before your doctor's visit. Even better—read a chapter to your doctor. This book is perfect for waiting rooms. Laughter is often the best medicine. Consider *Pet Goats & Pap Smears* medical foreplay for a fun office visit. In these pages you will discover how doctors think and why doctors suffer. I welcome you to develop a new level of appreciation for your physician.

## Teenagers

I didn't write this book for teenagers. But then a friend shared a story about her sixteen-year-old son. One afternoon he asked his mom, "Who is this Pamela Wible?"

"She's a friend and a doctor in town," his mom replied. "Why?"

"I see this doctor friend of yours on Facebook. She writes the coolest things about sex and penises!"

"What does she write?"

"I can't tell you all the details, Mom!"

Teenagers don't want to discuss penises with their parents. Exploring sexuality through medical adventure stories is more fun. *Pet Goats & Pap Smears* offers a nonjudgmental way for young adults to understand risky behaviors and learn how to protect themselves from sexually transmitted infections.

A healthy intimate relationship is always built on honesty. If you are a teenager reading this book, I hope to encourage you first to be honest with yourself, so that you can be true to your partner.

## People You Love

This is a gift book. Give this book to your best friends, your mothers, and daughters. Remind the women in your life to get their Pap smears—cervical cancer is preventable! Please give this book to teens and college students. *Pet Goats & Pap Smears* is perfect for book clubs, long car or plane rides, and is a great icebreaker for your next dinner party. Always keep a copy in your purse or your golf cart!

While you're reading, keep a list of loved ones you think may benefit from this book.

_____

_____

_____

_____

_____

_____

_____

_____

_____

# Author's Note

The stories in this book are true.

To my delight, most patients have asked that I use their real names and are eager to share their stories with the media. Others have requested anonymity, and their names have been changed. Occasionally, a story is a composite of more than one patient.

I have written these stories for the most part using present tense to help them come alive for you. Stories are meant to be shared with an open heart and mind. It is an honor to share them with you, and I invite you to share them with the important people in your life.

Storytelling is one of the most powerful ways we learn.

Read this book straight through or in sections—whatever inspires you. Medical students and doctors may want to reference the sections "On Joy" and "On Creativity" for inspiration between patient visits. The section "On Death" may be comforting after experiencing the loss of a patient. Consider reading chapters multiple times to explore the deeper meanings in the stories.

## Medical Disclaimer

Medical recommendations in this book are patient specific and are not meant for individual readers. Every person is unique. Please contact a medical professional to discuss your specific condition.

## Imagine . . .

While reading these stories, I encourage you to imagine what ideal medical care is for you. I invite you to partake in the Imagine exercises at the beginning and end of the book. And along the way, feel free to *doodle*!

# Imagine . . .

### Design . . . Draw . . . Dream . . . **Your Ideal Clinic** . . .

# Imagine . . .

### Design . . . Draw . . . Dream . . . **Your Ideal Doctor** . . .

# Pet Goats & Pap Smears™

## 101 Medical Adventures to Open Your Heart & Mind

Pamela Wible, M.D.

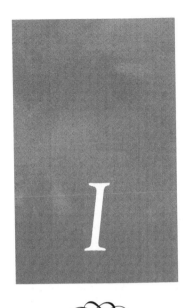

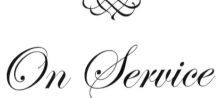

# On Service

How do I know if I've provided great service?
It's not from a patient satisfaction survey.
I can usually tell when I look out my office window
and see my fifty-year-old patient with pneumonia
skipping through the parking lot with her balloon.

# 1

# Town Hall Medicine

It's March 6, 2005. I'm greeting the residents of Lane County, Oregon, as they line up at the door. Housewives and hippies, bus drivers and business-men, artisans, farmers, and folks of all ages take their seats as I move to the front of the room.

I'm a thirty-seven-year-old unemployed physician. Burned out from the bureaucracy, I left assembly-line medicine because I'm not a robot and patients are not widgets. I'm done holding patients hostage on a conveyor belt. Today, I'm asking patients to lead.

I announce, "This afternoon, I invite you all to design an ideal clinic for our community. Not a clinic created by experts or lobbyists, politicians or physicians, but one created entirely by patients like you." And I promise, "I'll do whatever you want as long as it's legal." I turn on relaxing music, dim the lights, and continue, "I welcome you to imagine what it would feel like to walk into an ideal clinic in an optimal health care system."

Pages overflow with diagrams and doodles, poetry and prose as citizens introduce themselves and share their hopes and dreams.

Mimi, a free-spirited mother of two, recites, "An ideal clinic is a sanctu-ary, a safe place, a place of wisdom where we learn to live harmlessly, listen with empathy, observe without judgment. It's a place where a revolution starts, where we rediscover our priorities."

Lynette, a Chinese woman with an Australian accent, interjects, "No front counters separating people from people, complimentary massage while waiting, fun surgical gowns!"

Jacob, a soft-spoken guy with dreadlocks, imagines a clinic with

3

# Town Hall Medicine

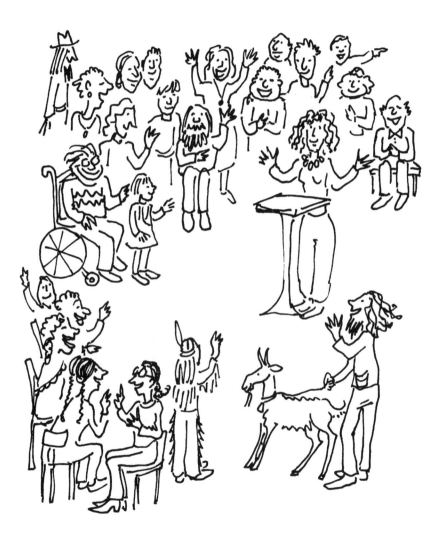

Patients create their own clinic.

"intriguing magazines and a pet cat that greets people at the door," plus "a big garden and a running stream where you come over for lunch and play with the pet goats who inadvertently heal your broken leg."

I'm inspired, but overwhelmed. I'm wondering how I will do it all. Maybe I'll teach the goat to give a massage. Then an Indian woman reassures, "Most importantly, the doctor would be someone with a big heart and a great love for people and service, someone whose presence itself is enough to cheer a patient."

In their words I rediscover myself.

From living rooms and Main Street cafés to yoga studios and neighborhood centers—nine town halls in six weeks—I collect 100 pages of submitted testimony. For the first time, my job description is written by *patients*, not administrators.

While I purchase equipment and negotiate contracts, I'm imagining the sanctuary filled with peaceful music. I smile as the clinic cat leads clients through a tunnel entrance to a Caribbean-themed exam room filled with beanbags and balloons. Finally, I see the place where nobody is turned away for lack of money, where the doctor answers the phone, says come right over, and is waiting when you arrive.

One month later we're open. Still looking for our pet goat.

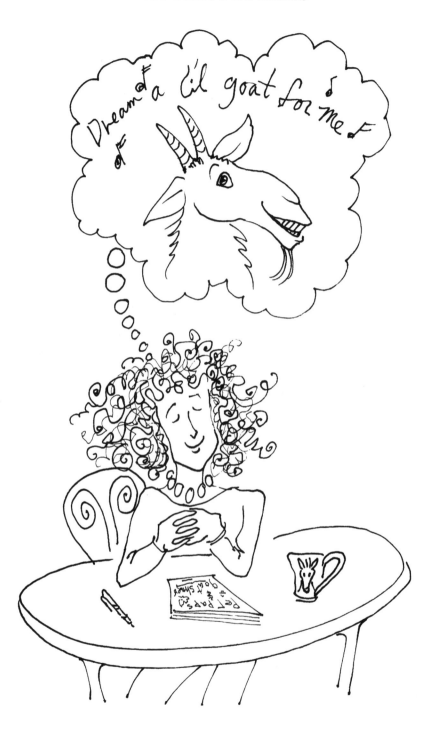

# 2

# Peanut Butter & Jacob

It's April 1, 2005—opening day for our clinic. I chose to open on April Fools' Day just in case my furniture didn't arrive in time. I imagined patients sitting on the floor in an empty clinic as I'd laugh, "April Fools!" But everything is here; the clinic is beautiful. I lean down, resting on my hands and knees, and kiss the floor. It seems surreal and so dusty down here.

The clinic—housed in a wellness center tucked into a wooded hillside—offers yoga, massage, and a solar-heated pool and hot tub. Forget sitting in a waiting room. Now patients may relax in a Jacuzzi. But there's never a wait. Appointments are on time—guaranteed—or patients may choose a present from a giant wicker basket by the door.

I'm arranging the gifts while waiting for patients, when a whisper lures me into the exam room.

"Doctor Pamela? Psssst. Hey, it's me, Jacob."

Outside the window is a skinny hippie dude with dreadlocks. I'm so excited. Here's my first patient—the town-hall guy who wants pet goats!

A twenty-five-year-old college student, Jacob is an artist, writer, street performer, and a free-spirited lover of life. He's uninsured and stops by for a quick blood pressure check before taking off for Japan in a few weeks.

Jacob lies down on the sofa and offers me a bite of his peanut butter and jelly sandwich as I open my laptop to gather his medical history. Immediately I'm swept up by his life's adventures—from his zany goat antics to his summer romance in Bangkok.

"Wait a minute," I interrupt. "Why are you here again?"

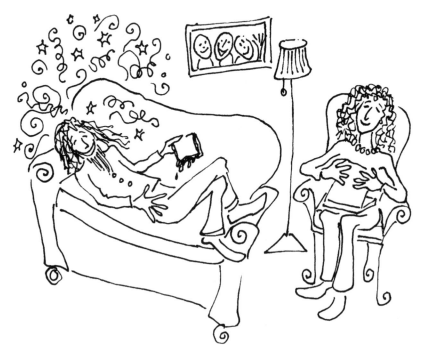

**Inside every patient is a storyteller.**

"Oh, at my college physical a few years ago they told me my pressure was kinda high."

"Do you remember how high?"

"Umm . . . like 160-over-something-like-100."

"So what did they do?"

"Oh, they weren't too concerned. My chiropractor thought maybe my alignment was off in my neck. I'm on Chinese herbs and a homeopathic. What do you think, Pamela?"

"Have you had any recent blood pressure checks?"

"Yesterday at the grocery store, the top number was 210. I think the bottom number was, like, 130-ish," Jacob says, before giving me a hand-painted invitation to his performance next week. "I'll be doing some puppetry, spoken word, and dance. You should come, Pamela."

"Okay, Jacob, but let's go into the exam room for a moment."

He tells me all about his puppets as I check his blood pressure and confirm the bad news. I'm terrified he'll have a stroke any minute, but I can't stop laughing as Jacob tells me about the chimichanga he ate for lunch last Tuesday. His comedic ramblings could be a sign of hypertensive brain damage or an April Fools' Day stunt.

I've got to focus. This is a life-or-death situation. I need to call his parents. Wait. Let me think. First, I'll order an ultrasound of his kidneys. But Jacob has his own plan of action.

"I've been told I have too much chi. I'm thinking I'll avoid peanut butter. What do you think of cutting back on peanut butter, Pamela?"

"According to the latest research, peanut butter restriction is not the best approach," I explain as I squeeze in next to him on the sofa.

Oblivious to the gravity of his condition, Jacob leads me through various dietary theories. "So I'm off soy sauce, Pamela, but I do still drink pickle juice right out of the jar, and I wonder if you think I should quit."

"Salt, soy sauce, and brine all raise your blood pressure, Jacob. Maybe quit the pickle juice and begin this medication. What do ya say?" I pat him on the shoulder and whisper, "Hey Jacob, your blood pressure is *really* high. Let's go to the hospital for some tests. I'll talk to your parents. Okay?"

After bantering back and forth for ten minutes, he agrees.

The next day, I bike downtown to the outdoor artisan fair where Jacob's family sells handmade hats. I meet with his dad, Jim. "Hey Jim. I'm Pamela. I'm Jacob's doctor. We've got a problem."

"Really?"

"Yep. Jacob's blood pressure is up to 210/130."

"Is that high?" Jim asks.

"Normal blood pressure is less than 120/80, so it's nearly double what it should be. He's on medication and I've ordered some tests."

The following week, Jacob's ultrasound reveals a narrowed artery to his right kidney. I accompany his family to the hospital and meet with the interventional radiologist who will be performing the angioplasty to open Jacob's artery. Turns out we trained at the same medical school in Texas!

I wave to Jacob from a window in the surgical radiology suite. While singing along to country music in the background, I watch Jacob's procedure on the monitor. The radiologist dilates Jacob's right renal artery with a balloon-tipped catheter to restore blood flow to his kidney.

That evening Jacob's blood pressure is normal with no medication. I celebrate with my own impromptu performance for Jacob and his family. I reenact Jacob's life-saving procedure, using his catheters and wires that I scavenged from the trash as souvenirs—perhaps props for his upcoming puppet show.

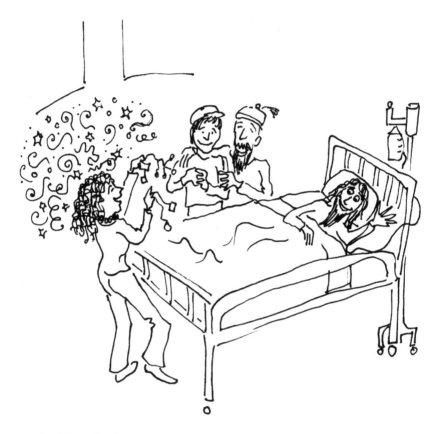

**Avoid medical jargon. Always speak the patient's language.**

What was this experience worth? For me, it was priceless. I waived my portion of the hospital bill. Jacob paid me ninety bucks, and his parents made me a beautiful hat.

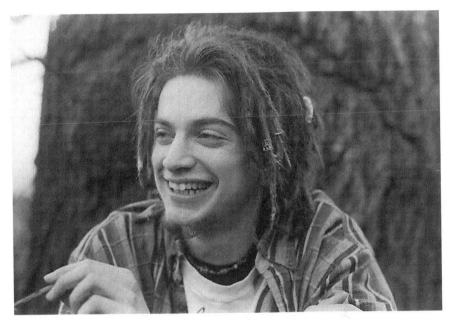

**Never miss an opportunity to save a patient's life.**

3

# Free Cancer Screening

Eric is an uninsured musician. He runs into me in a grocery store late one night. I'm trying to decide between organic low-fat pesto and gluten-free marinara, when he says, "Pamela, I think I've got cancer." He pauses. "It's this spot on my hand."

While grabbing the marinara, I glance over at his flat, little mole and say, "Nope, that's definitely not cancer." He spends the next five minutes chasing me around the store trying to pass me ten bucks. "Forget about it," I tell him. "I got my pasta sauce. You didn't slow me down at all."

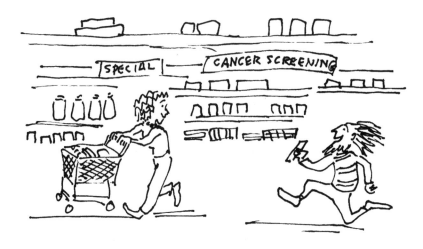

**Sometimes the best medicine is free!**

# 4

# Forget the ER, Try the Y

Although I choose to work part time, I'm available 24/7 for my patients.

One Saturday afternoon, Leslie calls to tell me her son has horrible poison oak. But I'm at my nephew Jordan's basketball game. So I say, "Meet me at the Y." Ten minutes later I'm treating her son right on the sidelines.

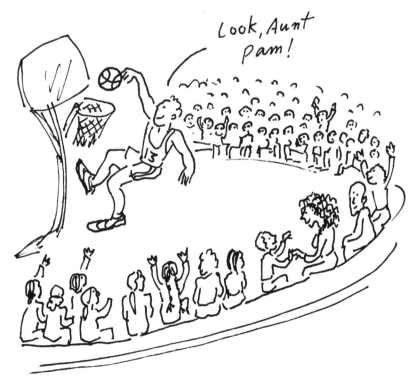

**Sometimes the best medicine is at the YMCA!**

# 5

# Forget the ER, Try the DMV

Rob, an uninsured carpenter, sliced off the tip of his finger last week. Now he worries it's infected. The ER is a few hundred bucks plus a long wait, so he gives me a call. My emergency cell rings as I'm pulling up to the Department of Motor Vehicles to renew my driver's license. Rob—an old friend and current patient—lives right around the corner, so I tell him, "Meet me at the DMV."

"Perfect!" he says. "I've got a car title to transfer. See ya in a few."

Minutes later he grabs a number and the seat beside me.

While we're waiting, I evaluate his finger.

"No infection. It's healing fine, Rob."

Just then my number is announced. As I make my way to the front of the room to pose for my photo, Rob tags along, celebrating his impromptu medical visit with anyone who will listen. Even the clerks behind the counter can't stop smiling.

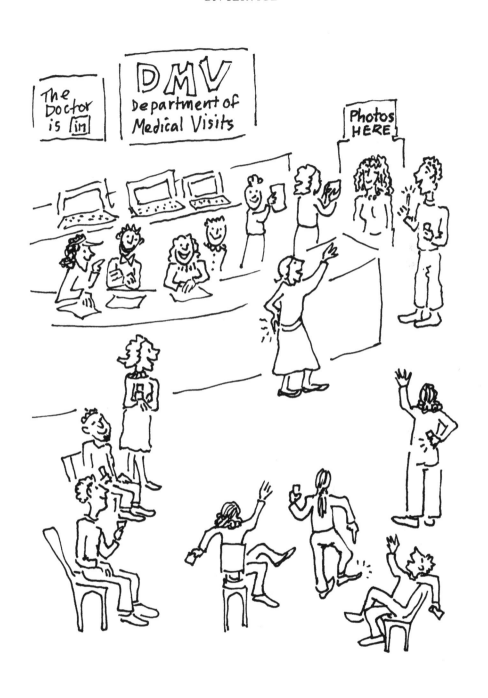

Sometimes the best medicine is at the DMV!

# 6

# A Health-Care Tip

I open a Christmas card from Dave and Lisa, and out falls a fifty-dollar check as a tip. All these years and I've never received a tip. Wow! Why now? The memo line reads, "For special care." I call to demand an explanation.

Dave answers.

"What did I do to deserve a tip?"

Dave explains, "Remember a few months back when we called you Friday at midnight? Lisa was in such distress. Within a few minutes you gave us guidelines on how to handle her breathing problems."

"Oh, I remember. Okay."

Dave's voice cracks. "After your call, I broke down in tears of thankfulness [as he's doing now]. If it hadn't been for you, we would have ended up in the ER and faced the additional stressors of 'Who are you? What's your insurance? Fill out this form.' And if that had been the case, I might have gone over the edge."

"Yes. I understand now."

"On top of all that, your courage to start an ideal medical clinic has inspired me to start my own recycled-furniture business. Like you, I want to be part of a solution instead of a passive contributor to a problem."

"Okay. Got it. Thanks."

Tips reward great service. I never cashed my first tip. It's in my box of cool souvenirs, along with the piece of bubble gum I shared with my high school boyfriend and the slip of paper from my recent fortune cookie that reads:

> You could make a name for yourself in the field of medicine.

# 7

# A Rich Stitch

While washing dishes, Dawn slices her pinky finger on broken glass. Bleeding through her dishcloth, she drives to the rural clinic down the road. As she pulls into their parking lot, she calls me. I reroute her to my office.

As I numb her finger for surgery, Dawn says, "I'm so relieved you came in on your day off. I was about to check in at the other clinic."

"Why didn't you just stay there?" I ask.

"A few months back, I was there for a cut on my head. I waited two hours with a bunch of sick people coughing, my head bleeding, rag in hand, and crying 'cause the darn thing hurt so bad."

"That sucks."

"It's just the nurse practitioner at the clinic. She's been there forever. She sewed up my forehead, practicing some new stitch on me. On my way out, they were surprised that I wanted to pay in full with cash. Then they charged me $600!"

"Practicing a new stitch on you? Maybe they should've paid *you* $600."

"They felt bad, said they didn't know I was uninsured. They would have known had they actually read the three-page form I filled out in the waiting room!"

"Did they give you a discount?"

"The nurse practitioner wanted to lower the bill, but she told me she just teamed up with a big medical group in town to stay afloat, so her hands were tied. How sad that she—of all people—had given in to all the bullshit. The worst part is I think she really cares. It used to be a real clinic."

I'm tying off the last stitch as Dawn concludes, "So 600-plus dollars later I'm back for suture removal. She's got the entire staff gathered around me to learn how to remove the special stitch. Maybe they *should have been* paying me."

I finish up, bandage her finger, and say, "That will be $800 for today." I pause. "Just kidding. Does $160 work for you?"

"How about $200?" Dawn says as she passes me a wad of twenties.

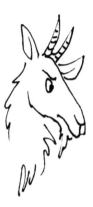

8

# Dental Floss

Michael is a welder and woodworker. Today he's here for migraines. Examining him, I notice some large scars on his arms and legs.

"So what's up with all the scars?" I ask.

"I've injured myself in construction accidents over the years. I'm uninsured and can't afford hospital bills, so I take care of things myself. This scar on my thigh is pretty bad. It tore open after I stitched it."

"You stitched yourself up? With what?" I ask.

"Dental floss."

"Wow! Do you use waxed or unwaxed? Cinnamon or mint? What an interesting idea, Michael. I've never heard of anyone flossing his legs."

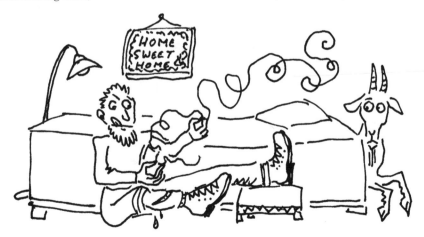

**Michael sews himself up with "accidental floss."**

# 9

# You Wanna Pay?

My mom and I are at her doctor's office. On our way out of the clinic, we stop at the front desk. Mom says, "I'd like to pay my bill."

The receptionists look baffled.

"You want to pay your bill?" one asks.

Mom is hard of hearing, so she raises her voice. "I'd like to pay my bill, please."

"You want to pay your bill?" asks the lead receptionist.

She leans forward and says a little louder, "Yes, I want to pay my bill now."

"She wants to pay now," says one of the receptionists to the next.

Mom's frustration has become visible. She pulls out her wallet and yells, "What kind of service is this? I want to pay now!" as she slams a few hundreds on the counter. "Cash!" she shouts.

The receptionists talk among themselves. Then the lead receptionist gets up from her chair. "I'll need to get the clinic manager."

"We'll just have to check with the doctor and make sure it's okay," another adds.

Mom looks around at all the patients—with their canes, walkers, and wheelchairs—packed into the waiting room, and then looks again at the receptionists and shouts, "What's going on? Doesn't anyone pay their bills around here?"

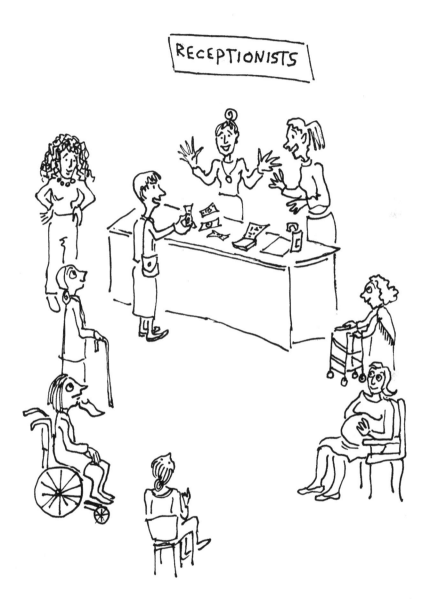

**Insurance-dominated health care turns a paying patient into a medical oddity.**

# 10

# On His Nerves

Kevin, an uninsured landscaper, calls for an appointment. "Doc, remember the lumps on my arm? I'd like you to remove them."

"Sure. No problem." I schedule him for an extended surgical visit.

When he arrives, I examine his arm. "Kevin, you've got benign fatty tumors on top of a nerve in your forearm. These lumps don't really need to be removed. It's a risky surgery. Plus, I don't want to paralyze your arm."

Kevin agrees not to proceed with the surgery, but then he starts ranting about a previous physician. "This guy didn't listen, never even looked me in the eyes, didn't act like he even cared! What's with all these rich, arrogant doctors these days?"

We sit down and I explain, "Physicians are good people who are victimized. They're overwhelmed and exhausted." I look straight into Kevin's eyes. "It starts in school with dehumanizing and barbaric animal experiments. Everyone in my medical school class had to kill a dog to graduate! Add the sleepless nights on call and the economic stranglehold. Do you realize med students graduate with over $200,000 in student loans? Then, when they graduate they're funneled into assembly-line clinics. After all the abuse, doctors are emotionally and spiritually disconnected from themselves and their patients. It's tragic. No wonder we lose a doctor each day to suicide and sixty percent of doctors want to quit."

I pause to inhale.

Kevin is quiet.

"Here's the problem: I didn't do anything, so I have no idea what to charge you."

Kevin stands up and empties everything from his pockets. On the table are some crunched-up dollar bills, some coins, and some pocket lint. He gives me $87.23 for something I can't even put into words.

I think he paid me for being human.

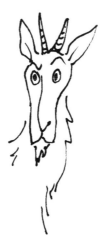

# 11

# Time Is Money

Meet Elaine.

We lost touch for a few years, but today she catches up with me. Like most girlfriends, we share adventures of love, travel, and work.

"What have you been up to?" she asks.

"I left assembly-line medicine. Now I help patients create their own clinics. I'm always looking for innovative ideas."

"Here's one for you: I get frustrated waiting at doctors' offices. One day I decided to stop being frustrated and do something about it."

"So what did you do?"

"While working as a consultant for Boeing, I had a midday appointment in Seattle. My doctor left me in the waiting room for ninety minutes! So I billed him for my waiting time at my $47.00 hourly rate."

"That's wild. I've never heard of patients billing doctors."

"I'm not looking to make money off doctors. I'm simply trying to recoup lost wages. A bill sends the message that my time is not free. I've sent six invoices to date, and half of them were paid."

"Elaine, that's amazing."

"Yes, and it's not specific to medicine. When the cable guy tells me to wait at home for three hours, I inform him: 'Expect a $141.00 bill. Is that okay with your boss?' So we compromise—the driver agrees to call fifteen minutes ahead of his arrival, and I agree to meet him at my house."

"I'm impressed. You really stand up for yourself."

As I reflect on our conversation, I realize Elaine values herself and her time. I wonder who else bills for wait time? Cab drivers charge for waiting.

Restaurants may provide discounted meals for the inconvenience. Airlines cover hotel rooms for undue delays. . . .

Scheduled patients deserve prompt service, but what's a delayed doctor to do? Some physicians apologize. Others give gifts. I offer handmade soap. A doc in Seattle gifts Starbucks cards, and one in Southern California provides movie passes to postponed patients.

In Dallas, one doc—who canceled his appointments for a family emergency—gave each patient fifty bucks for the inconvenience. He says, "It's only fair. My patients' time is just as valuable—if not more so—than mine."

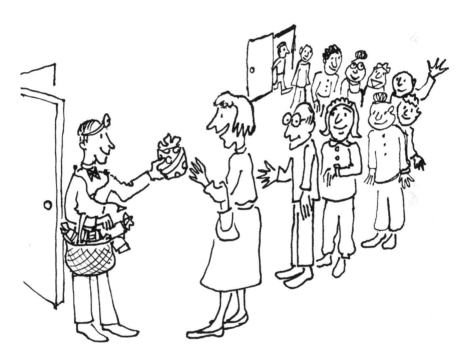

**Delayed doctor doles out door prizes.**

P.S. While writing this book, I forgot to show up for a patient's appointment. We rescheduled for a few days later. When she entered the office, I handed her a fifty-dollar bill and explained, "It's my policy to charge fifty dollars for no shows. I'm happy to hold myself to the same standard."

# 12

# Soap Opera

Beside my office door is a big wicker basket. Inside are local, handmade specialty soaps, lotions, and lip balms. If I'm more than ten minutes late for an appointment, patients pick a gift.

Last year, my gift-giving routine was picked up by CNN as a national news story. Then came calls from morning show producers at other major networks. I passed along the names of several doctors who are doing the same thing.

Nine months later, I get a call from yet another news agency. A reporter from Manhattan wants to interview a patient. Good timing. Today, I'm running late due to a complicated case, so my last patient got a gift! I call her. "Kerry, you got a bar of soap today out of the gift basket, right?"

"Yes! Thank you so much. I've been carrying it around with me all day. It smells great. I love it!" she exclaims.

"A reporter would like to talk to you about the soap."

"What?"

"A reporter from Manhattan is doing a story on doctors who give gifts to patients when they run late. He'd like to interview you."

"Really? Me?"

"Would that be okay?" I ask.

"On TV? A reporter from New York City wants to interview me on television? About my bar of soap?" Kerry asks.

"No, not on TV. He wants to interview you on the phone for an article," I explain.

"About my bar of soap?"

"Yep! I guess it's a national news story when doctors respect patients' time."

"Okay. Sure, I'll do it," she laughs.

And so Kerry, a housewife, makes headlines when she tells the big-city reporter all about her organic bar of chamomile-lavender, goat's-milk soap. "My husband won't let me buy that handmade soap," she adds, "because it's too expensive."

What does she think about gifts from her doctor?

Kerry gets on her soapbox. "I've always been low on the totem pole," she says. "I never had any authority. It's so much more fair and respectful to acknowledge that my time is valuable, too."

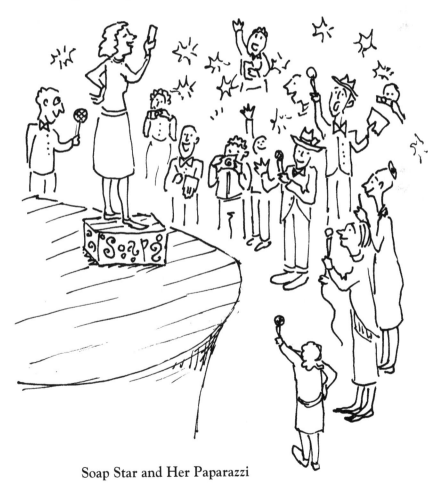

**Soap Star and Her Paparazzi**

# 13

## My Favorite Prescriptions

Patients expect prescriptions, and doctors deliver. The problem is, what most patients need can't be delivered in a little pink pill. During the past twenty years, I've written a lot of prescriptions. Here are my favorites:

Have great sex three times per week!
Take a vacation to the coast.
Go on a seven-day silent retreat in the woods.
Find a girlfriend!
Quit your job!
Reconnect with deceased relatives.
Have your husband do the dishes for a week.
Go on a media fast for a month.
Stop worrying.
Fall in love with yourself.
Have your children massage your feet before bed.
Speak your truth.
Get a puppy.
Write a book.
Come with me to a writers' conference. I'll pay.
See an energy healer. I'll go with you.
Get an exorcism.
Sell your car and commute by bike.
Avoid your mother-in-law.

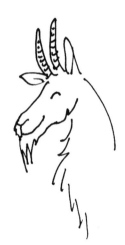

Maybe people don't need so many medical appointments. Most people just need to relax, have fun, and hang out at a petting zoo.

# 14

# A Human Fax

Carol is a forty-four-year-old black woman with asthma, high cholesterol, low thyroid, fibromyalgia, arthritis, and migraines. Since her only daughter was murdered last year, she has had severe insomnia that can lead to hallucinations if left untreated. She smokes, but says she's cutting back. A self-admitted chocoholic, she uses sugar to ease her emotional pain. Carol suffers from anxiety, depression, and PTSD as a result of multiple sexual assaults that began with childhood incest, followed by date rape as a teen, and then a lifetime of domestic abuse.

Today, Carol comes in with atypical chest pain and needs an urgent cardiac evaluation, but due to her abuse history she refuses to see male physicians. The problem is, there is only one female cardiologist in our entire county. I plead her case on the official referral form, but I'd like to bypass the bureaucracy.

Instead of faxing the referral to a mysterious fax machine, I ride my bicycle to the health plan's administrative office. As I enter, the secretary stops me. "May I help you?"

"I'm Dr. Wible. Here with a fax."

As she attempts to retrieve it, I pull back. Maybe if *I* were this fax, then I could finally see what goes on in these windowless referral processing centers.

"Take me to this fax machine," I say, pointing to the fax number on the form.

She asks me to sign in and hands me a temporary badge. Then she unlocks a pair of doors and leads me into a huge room full of cubicles. We make our way through a maze of carpeted corridors, and she deposits me at the fax machine in the corner.

"But now where do I go?" I ask. "Who would pick me up from this tray?"

"Follow me," she says.

We turn left and she drops me off in Connie's cubicle. Connie looks up at me in my bicycle garb. Few physicians frequent Connie's cubicle, and those who do are usually not wearing bike shorts, a helmet, and glitter. She seems to enjoy the attention.

I hand her the fax, provide a synopsis of Carol's case, and then ask, "So how do you know if I'm approved?"

Connie clicks her mouse three times and announces, "You're approved!"

As I'm preparing to leave, she promises, "Dr. Wible, from now on your referrals will always be approved!"

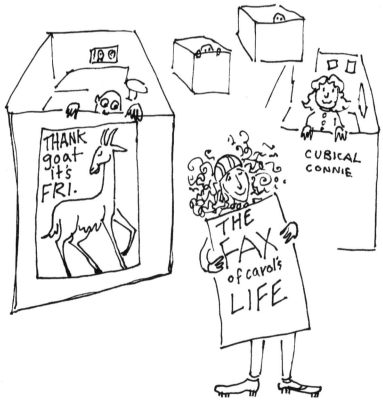

**Though technology is often revered as health care's panacea, never underestimate the power of a human fax.**

# 15

# My Favorite Hospital CEO

One day I get a call from Steve, the sixty-year-old CEO of a hospital system. "We'd like you to help us replicate your ideal clinic model in our hospitals. Do you think it's possible here in the Midwest?"

"Absolutely. It's time to let patients lead. I'm happy to help."

During our hour-long conversation, we agree to work together.

"You've opened my mind and heart to so many things," Steve says. "I'm very excited that you'll be coming to our community and helping our doctors become happier practitioners. I really think this is divinely inspired. God bless you."

The hospital system is Catholic, and its mission is to serve the underprivileged. So I ask that we visit with the Amish and Hmong, the children and elderly, the poor and suffering. And we listen to their hopes and dreams as we invite them to create their ideal hospitals.

Over a forty-eight-hour period, I lead nine small sessions, plus two community luncheons with 300 people each. As Steve walks to the podium, I whisper, "Remember: don't speak like a CEO. Speak from your heart."

"Will do," he says.

After a welcoming prayer, Steve says, "Today, I'm sharing something I've never shared publicly, but Dr. Wible is making me do it. It's difficult for me." He pauses. "My son, Nick, died of a brain tumor when he was eight. He was sick for five years. We were at the best hospitals in the country. Nick got wonderful care from doctors, but his care between surgeries was terribly insulting and disrespectful. He was treated like a number. Nurses would come into the room laughing and talking about their vacations while

I'm watching my son die. So much anger built up in me and my wife. After Nick died, I made a vow to myself that, as a hospital administrator, I would ensure people are treated decently."

The room is still.

"Today," Steve continues, "we're asking you to take control of our health system. We want to empower our community to dream about what our hospitals could be. And then we want to make it happen. We are here to serve you. We want to understand, from you, how to do this."

As I take the stage, I hug Steve and whisper, "You did it."

The lights dim in the ballroom.

Our visioning process begins: "I welcome you to close your eyes and imagine walking into your ideal hospital. Notice how it feels. See the colors, textures. How does your hospital serve the community?"

People pass the microphone and share their visions: "A hospital is energetically sound, every nail pounded with love . . . it's a place that feels like home . . . where families can be close . . . where there is hands-on healing . . . waterfalls, warm floors, essential oils . . . with prayer and God's loving light . . . it's a place where a sick person does not feel alone . . . where fears are addressed . . . and life and death are embraced with grace."

I glance at Steve. He gives me a thumbs up. We smile at each other as the next woman stands.

"When my goat was sick, my vet came right out to my farm with her six-year-old son," she shares. "We all chased the goat down in the pasture and she took care of him in the barn. She went on to the nesting box to care for a new litter of kittens and then set up a triage table on the front porch for our house cat. All to the cost of a thirty-five-dollar house call! That's what I want!" she concludes. "Not to be treated like a human, but like a goat!" Laughter echoes throughout the room.

A teenage boy jumps up and grabs the microphone. "Can I get a massage and more kids to share my room so it won't be so lonely, and a walk-through garden on the roof so we can have fresh food?"

"Can I have dinosaur books by my bed?" a small boy asks.

Just then, a young schoolgirl exclaims, "I want a big mural on the outside of the hospital showing people who are having fun! Plus zoo animals and aquariums everywhere, and a glass floor with fish swimming by."

# Town Hall Medicine

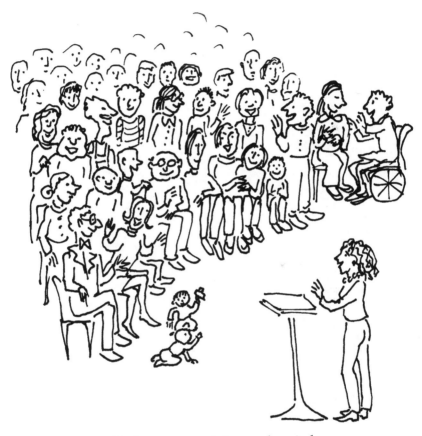

**Patients create their own hospital.**

I look over at Steve. He's sitting in his chair, eyes closed, taking slow, deep breaths. I recall Steve telling me that if his son, Nick, were alive, he'd probably be a teacher. "God sends only good," Steve had shared. "Nick was part of my lesson in this world. He volunteered to do it. We will never know why."

I sense his son, Nick, in the room. He's teaching us that it's okay to be human, that we can heal a child even without saving his life. And that a son can heal a father just by opening his heart.

Maybe the most profound healing happens when we are fully present for one another, in community, outside the hospital walls.

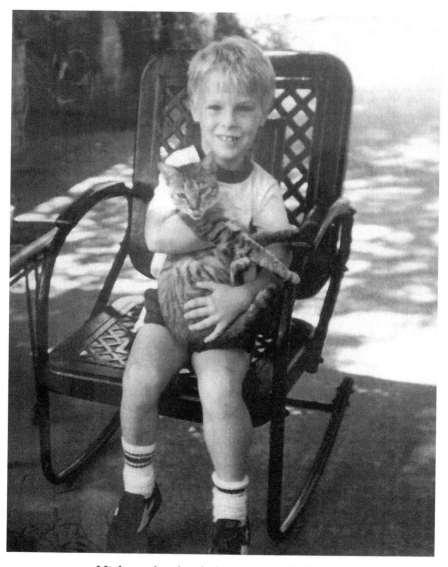

**Nick teaches his father to open his heart.**

# 16

# Amish Sense

Phoning isn't an option. Nor is e-mail. So I write a letter to the head elder, asking that the Amish community meet with me. He agrees.

Today is the day. I accompany Steve, the hospital CEO, to an Upper Midwest town so tiny that the post office is inside the grocery store. On the third floor of a local bank, we open the door to an empty conference room. But when we flip on the lights, we discover twelve bearded Amish men in straw hats. They are wearing matching black work boots, navy blue pants, shirts, and zip-up jackets. The men are seated, evenly spaced from eldest to youngest in a slight semicircle.

My first thought is that maybe I shouldn't be wearing a short skirt with a low-cut blouse.

I smile, introduce myself, and begin: "We're here today to serve you, to listen to your dreams, your visions of ideal health care."

No response.

I lean forward. "How can we help you be comfortable in the hospital?"

Silence.

I wait.

They sit quietly.

I stare at them.

They stare at me.

Then an elder says, "We're comfortable now."

After thirty minutes, I'm still trying to get a dialogue going. "Please tell us your views on health, disease, death."

No reaction.

"Okay then, I'll tell you about me. I'm a family doc from Oregon. I got tired of pushing patients around, so I held town hall meetings to ask people what they want. You know what people want? They want to go back to the 1950s when you could walk to the doctor's office in the neighborhood."

All at once, all the men smile the same little smile. I don't know exactly why they are smiling. But what I'm doing must be working, so I keep rambling along in my usual, animated style with lots of hand gestures. A moment later they burst into laughter. What did I say that made them laugh?

I'm noticing that these Amish men react in unison. They all smile at the exact same time. When they laugh, they all laugh at the same instant, and now they're all staring at me with big, beautiful smiles. And they begin to share their lives with me.

"We like to pay our bills," the head elder states. "We collect door to door in our community. Families contribute what they can, but sometimes the hospital won't take our money. We don't want charity care. We want to pay our fair share."

One man pulls out a piece of paper. "This is the bill for my son's surgery. He injured his arm. Had a simple surgery. Took an hour. They charged us for two anesthesiologists. Did my son need two anesthesiologists?"

"That's a good question," I reply.

The CEO reaches over for the bill and explains, "With the new health care laws, you'll be covered by insurance."

"To have health insurance means one doesn't trust in God," an elder states. "What we request is a fair bill."

"Yes, that's what Americans want: a fair bill," I add.

I look at the CEO and suggest, "Let's give fifty percent off at the door for anyone religiously opposed to lawsuits."

"I'll work on it," he says.

Now all the Amish men want to tell their stories.

"If we have a child in the hospital with a burn," a young man shares, "we find burdock leaves prevent the need for skin grafts."

All the men nod in unison.

"I eat burdock root," I reply, "but I've never used the leaves."

We all smile.

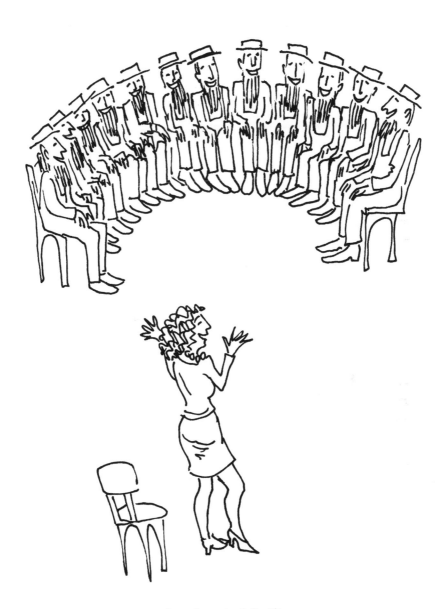

Synchronized Smiling

Another man says, "We like hospitals that respect our use of medicines that we find helpful."

"That makes sense. Do hospitals honor your wishes?" I ask.

"Some do."

"Where do you go?"

"To Ohio," says the head elder.

"Really? All the way to Ohio?"

"For my wife's gallbladder surgery, we loaded our family on the train to Ohio," explains a short, middle-aged man. "The hospital there is seventy percent cheaper."

"I know physician reimbursement is lower in Ohio," I acknowledge. "I guess that works to your advantage. But we want to serve you here at home so you won't need to take the train out of state."

After two hours, I stand up and approach the twelve men. One by one, I shake their hands. "It was such an honor to meet you all. Thank you for allowing me to be here."

The first gentleman looks up. "So you're moving here to be our doctor?"

"No, I'm going home to Oregon."

"You're not moving here to be our doctor?" another man begs.

"I wish I could be your doctor." I pause, hold his hand, and smile. "But I'm helping doctors all over the country to be the kind of doctors people want."

As we're driving away, the CEO exclaims, "I've never seen the Amish open up like that. I think they were ready to build you a buggy and move you into the neighborhood!"

# 17

# Letters to My Father

I've written many letters to my father. But there's a letter to my father that I'll never forget. And it wasn't from me.

The story begins the year I work alongside Steve on the executive team of his Midwest hospitals. Steve has hired me to bring community-designed health care to the region. I'm training hospital staff and leading town halls throughout the state to help citizens design their ideal hospitals.

During the project, my dad becomes ill. Death seems near. Steve asks to write a letter to my father. The request seems odd, but I pass along my father's address.

A week later, Dad calls. "Do you know a man named Steve?"

"I'm working with him. Why?"

"Today I received a very interesting letter from Steve." Dad reads aloud from Steve's letter:

> I find that, frequently, people are seen in different roles and their loved ones are sometimes among the last to know of their professional stature. My job requires attending a lot of funerals, and a theme I often hear is that we wait too long to express our gratitude. As the president of a health system, a father, and one who has lived long enough to appreciate what is truly important, I want to share my appreciation with you for being the father of such a tremendous physician and human being.

I feel tears rolling down my cheeks as Dad continues reading from Steve's letter:

> The world is often just a veil of tears and suffering. It is individuals like your daughter who are saints and examples to the rest of us. It frankly has been an answer to a prayer that your daughter has come to the people of our region, bringing hope and healing. Thank you for sharing her with us. Take care and God bless you.

"This is a remarkable letter," Dad says.

Steve is a remarkable man. I'd like to write a letter to Steve's father, but his father died. Even though I can't mail it, I still write my letter:

> As a physician who has worked for many clinics, hospitals, and health systems, I want to share my appreciation with you for being the father of such a courageous CEO. In a sea of self-serving CEOs, your son stands out as a man who leads from his heart. Steve has been an answer to a prayer, and I thank you for bringing him into the world and for sharing him with me.

Halfway through our project, Steve and the hospital system part ways.

Months later, I'm still sad that our collaboration ended prematurely. I e-mail Steve to ask how he feels.

"It's been tough," he replies. "I've been struggling. Because I am a man, it is challenging for me to get in touch with my feelings. So I had to reference my book on feeling words. I now realize that my initial feeling was one of surprise, followed shortly by grief. I don't buy into permanency. The death of my child was a lesson in detaching from loss with love."

Steve continues, "My staff and I had just completed our most successful year. I felt disheartened the way it all ended. There was no wrongdoing. We had seized the moment and were engaging our community in a real way. We were building trust and momentum. But now I feel liberated."

After reading Steve's e-mail, I phone him. "Steve, tell me about your ideal job."

"My ideal job," Steve shares, "is to be where God wants me. I want to apply my wisdom and expertise to serve people with cutting-edge programs that are meaningful and sustainable. I want to be with people who are not just trying to maximize short-term profits. I'd like to recruit doctors and see them happy. And live in a place I could call home. My ideal job will find me after I've done the necessary work to network and declare my dream. Thanks for your guidance and please know how grateful I am for our friendship."

Words shape our destiny.

A single word can hurt or heal. Well-chosen words can heal a single patient or an entire health system. And the right words will manifest an ideal job for Steve. Maybe the wise words of a hospital CEO helped my father make a full recovery.

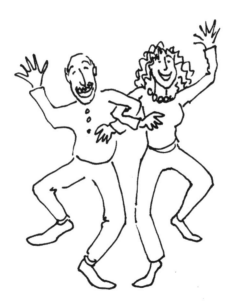

**Yep! Dad is out of the hospital and doing great!**

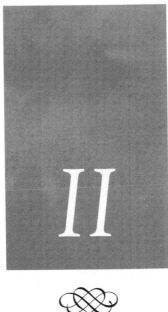

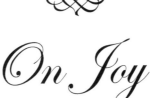

# On Joy

*If I'm not having fun at work, please send me home.*

# 18

# Child Labor

I'm often asked, "How can we bring more joy into medicine?"

Here's a quick solution: bring kids to work. When I was little, I accompanied my dad to the clinic, hospital, and morgue. It was so much fun! And I think people enjoyed having me there.

Now my friend, Amy, has kids volunteering in her clinic.

"How's that going?" I ask.

"My medical assistant's eight-year-old daughter is here most afternoons," Amy shares. "She restocks lab slips and waters the plants. She's a gorgeous, petite child, a very hard worker, and she follows directions well."

"What do your patients think of her?"

"She helps kids pick toys out of the toy box, and adults love having her around. In fact, yesterday I was draining a knee and injecting steroids into this big guy who was probably seven times her size. He was really scared. She tagged along and volunteered to hold his hand during the procedure. Afterward, she gave him a lollipop. It was so sweet."

I'm thrilled that my colleagues are bringing kids to work.

One doc tells me, "My newborn is working the front desk!"

"How the heck do ya do that? What does she do?" I ask.

"She shakes her rattle in her rocker, coos, and greets patients as they arrive. They love it!"

CHECK IN THERE.

# 19

# Laughing Out Loud

Lydia, a well-dressed brunette in her forties, limps in with heel pain. I introduce myself and we begin chatting. She hops up on the exam table and removes her sock. Her naked foot now rests on the edge of the table, just a few inches from my face.

Though we've never met before, we're joking the entire visit like girlfriends at a slumber party. Lydia tells me about the nutcase she met on an upscale dating site. I'm laughing so hard that I nearly inhale the navy-blue sock lint from between her toes.

After she leaves, I realize I never examined her foot! I call to apologize and offer an appointment free of charge. But she claims her pain disappeared.

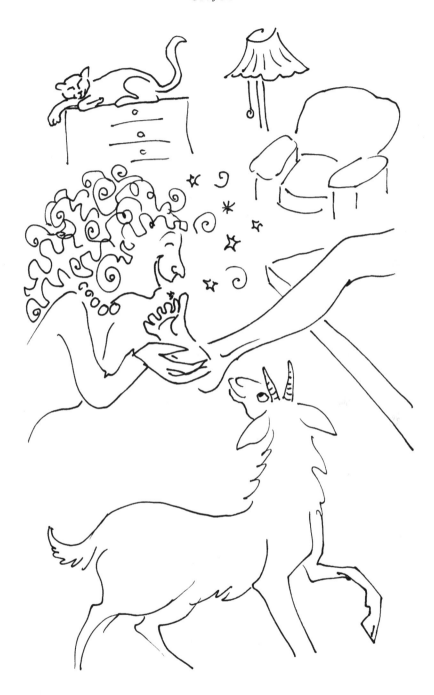

**Sometimes laughter *is* the best medicine.**

# 20

# A Fun Physician

"What would make going to the doctor fun?" I ask, interviewing people as I wander around the country. From San Francisco to Philadelphia and random spots in between, here's how Americans describe fun health care:

Doctor is excited, enthusiastic.
Bringing my dog with me.
Random trivia. Sharing fun facts about how the body works.
A game where you win a prize.
A trampoline. Juggling. Balloons.
Doctor is a stand-up comic who starts each session with a joke.
A waiting room with a hot tub.
Start each visit with a dance—something simple and fun.
I'm not looking for fun. It doesn't compute.
Good fun games. If the doctor is singing!
Doctors would give ME money when I show up!
The nurse is in a hot uniform.
Free medical marijuana.
Leave with a recipe, rather than a pill.
Doctor says, "You're in perfect health. See you in a year."
Partying. Music. Dancing. Blowing bubbles.
A food buffet, facial, and spa.
Deleting long, technical words.
On-site garden.
I'd be laughing the whole time.

A waitress at a small café adds: "Fun begins with a warm relationship, where you feel like you love and care about your doctors and they love and care about you. That creates all kinds of freedom to ask questions and bring up issues, to come up with insights—a complete human relationship."

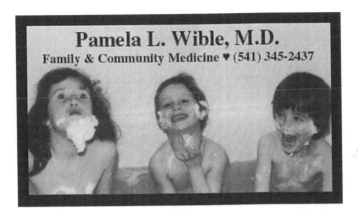

**Always have a fun business card.**

Hahaha! When my mom snapped this photo of me, my cousin Walter, and my brother Fred in the bathtub, she had no idea I would end up using it as my business card.

# 21

# Secret Santa & the Chlamydia Clown

It's December 2001. Time for Secret Santa: a clinic tradition in which employees are randomly assigned an office mate to whom they anonymously give gifts for the month.

The game is voluntary, and every year the male doctors choose not to participate. I approach Mike, the senior physician, and ask, "Hey, why don't you guys wanna do Secret Santa?"

"We used to," Mike says, "but we always forgot to give gifts. We'd end up with gals at the front desk crying during the holidays. Not a great morale booster."

I'm Jewish, so I'm not a natural at the Secret-Santa thing, but I love a great game. My Secret Santa already made some deliveries. I got a box of chocolates today. Last week a teddy bear was sitting on my charts. He was holding a singing card.

I'm Tracey's Secret Santa. She's eight months pregnant. Maybe I'll get her some cool baby stuff. Oh, I've got a better idea! I'll hire a clown to entertain Tracey at lunch. I clear my plan with the clinic manager. It's a go!

I'm not sure how to find a clown, so I grab the Yellow Pages, and just past "Clinics" is a quarter-page list of "Clowns."

I call the first clown. "I'd like to hire you."

"I've got a one-hour minimum, lady," he replies.

"Clowns have hourly minimums?" I pause. "I'm sure I can keep a clown busy for an hour."

I think to myself, I'll start with a prank on Mike. I just need the clown to pretend to have a sexually transmitted infection.

"I'd like you to come to a medical clinic."

"Nope. I only do children's parties."

I call the next clown. "I need a clown to come to our medical clinic."

"What do you need?" the clown asks.

"I'd like you to play a few jokes on people; maybe you could pretend to have gonorrhea."

"I'm a Christian clown, lady. I can't do that."

I learn most clowns in town are Christian and they don't feel comfortable having sexual infections. Plus, most clowns just do kids' parties. But I'm not giving up hope. I call every clown. Now I'm down to the last clown. "Hey, I need a clown to come to my medical clinic."

"Okay," she says. "I have a one-hour minimum."

"How much?" I ask.

"Seventy-five dollars."

"Great! But can you entertain the staff and patients with balloons and dancing? Oh, and can you pretend to have chlamydia? I want to play a prank on one of the doctors."

"I'm a Christian clown," she says.

Uh-oh. I'm worried she'll back out too. But she explains, "I work for Jesus. I'll do anything to make people happy."

"Awesome!" I review my instructions with her. We're set for Friday.

It's Friday. At noon, a short woman in baggy, pink-and-orange clothes and a huge, purple Afro arrives at the front desk. The secretary asks for her insurance. Another receptionist, with a serious case of clown phobia, suddenly runs to the back and hides. Meanwhile, Mike's nurse and I escort the clown to the exam room.

We wrap a sheet around the clown's midsection and she jumps up on the exam table. We guide her giant, pink circus shoes into the stirrups. Then the nurse yells down the hall: "Dr. Mike—we've got an emergency in Room 3!"

I hide behind the door. As Mike rushes into the room, the clown, on cue, sits straight up on the exam table and screams, "I thought it was gonna be a girl doctor!"

I figured Mike would laugh, but he's very serious. He tries to talk the clown down.

"Dr. Mike, she's scared she's got chlamydia," the nurse explains.

"Okay," Mike says, "just put your feet in the stirrups and let me examine you, miss."

The clown jumps off the table, pushes Mike to the side and runs down the hall with the sheet billowing behind her.

Mike's face is red. He can hardly speak. I hold his hand and walk him back to his office. Dazed, he stares up at me from his swivel chair and mumbles incoherently.

I put my hand on his shoulder. "Mike, remember Secret Santa?"

"Yes."

"I hired a clown. She had a one-hour minimum."

"You got me," Mike laughs.


Wait! Where's the clown? I still have thirty minutes left. There she is, inflating balloons in the lab. Since I'm Tracey's Secret Santa, I instruct the clown to chase Tracey around the clinic for the rest of the hour. Before the clown leaves, she teaches the male doctors to line dance down the hall and then leads a sing-along in the waiting room. Patients love it!


Later I reflect on the day's events. I now realize that when a clown claims to have chlamydia, the physician is obligated to take the clown very seriously. Patients can arrive for medical care in any costume they like. I guess not all clowns are clowning around. So the last joke was on me!

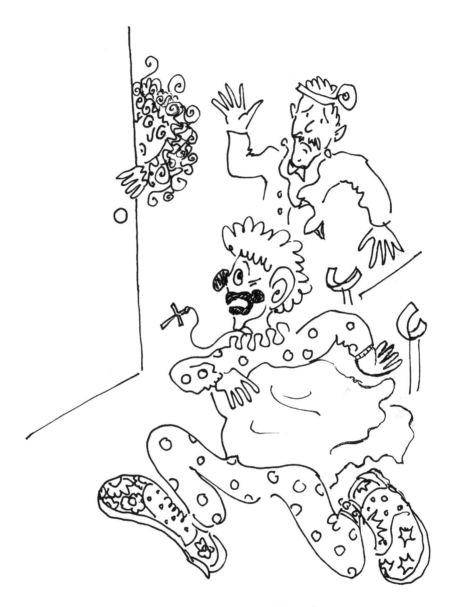

Even clowns can catch chlamydia.

# 22

# My Uncle Morty

It's Christmas season 2009. Mary Joy, a registered nurse, arrives for her appointment in a Santa hat. She needs a note signed for work.

"Pamela, I just heard your interview on NPR! Hey, I want to buy two more books. Can you autograph one to my daughter Sabrina?"

I sign the books and pass them to Mary Joy.

"I can't believe you wrote a book with Michelle Obama! Pamela, how can you do it all?"

"I get my passion from Uncle Morty. But I didn't know him too well, because he died when I was young."

"Was he a doctor?" she asks.

"Nope. He was a jazz pianist, a lawyer, and a consumer activist. He accompanied Billie Holiday at New York's Paramount Theater and wrote the lyrics and music for one of her songs. My family is in show business. My grandfather—Morty's dad—was a big theatrical-union leader and we're related to the Three Stooges!"

Mary Joy laughs.

"As an attorney, Morty looked out for the little guy. In the 1940s, he lost forty-six cents in bubble gum machines in the New York Subway stations. He sued in small-claims court and won! The judge called him an 'incurable optimist' and *Newsweek* recognized him as 'a hero to the frustrated.'"

"Forty-six cents is definitely a small claim!" she says.

"Look, Mary Joy, here's the article! My dad just mailed me this package full of information about Uncle Morty."

We look through the cardboard box filled with newspaper clippings.

Mary Joy finds a note from my dad and reads it aloud: "I'm sending some articles on my brother, Morty. There are such similarities in your battles with the status quo—the maladies of our society. Maybe you can use a quote one day in a book."

We dump the articles on the table and sort through them. Together we learn about my uncle. Morton Krouse grew up in Philadelphia. He studied consumer fraud and worked for a Philadelphia law firm. He applied for a consumer protection job with the city, but they turned him down because he was overqualified. So Morty donated his time to consumer advocacy. He did three radio shows every week and was a crusader for patients' rights.

He launched the American Patients Association to give patients a voice, improve care, and stop the "unbelievable overcharging by physicians." He wrote a booklet, *How to Cut Your Medical Bills in Half*. He founded Train More Doctors Society, Inc., testified before congressional committees in Washington, D.C., and educated state legislators on methods for doubling medical school enrollments.

Thumbing through the papers, we find a letter of commendation from Ralph Nader, and a page about Morty in *People* magazine. Underneath is a May 3, 1977, *Philadelphia Inquirer* article entitled, "27 Years Dedicated to Consumer and Krouse Is Getting Discouraged." The piece begins:

> There he was, Morton Krouse, 59, who describes himself as 'fat and friendly,' picketing the American Medical Association convention here last December and holding a sign that read: 'AMA Rips Off Consumer.' On occasion he would break into song—to the tune of *Santa Claus Is Coming to Town*: 'You better watch out, don't you get ill, you'll feel much worse when you get the bill. The AMA is coming to town.'

I parade around the room. "Uncle Morty did look like Santa!"
We keep reading.
Morty tells the reporter: "I'm trying to shock these doctors out of their smug, self-satisfied, money-making world and get them to return to healing."

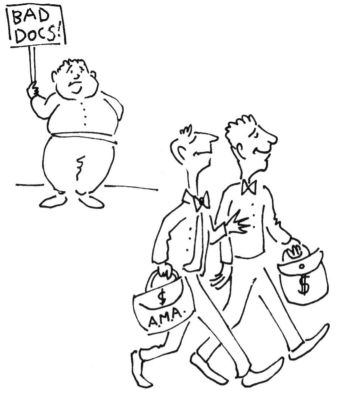

Mary Joy stands up and starts ranting. "I work with doctors every day. Why are they still so darn condescending and disrespectful? It's insane. Patients and staff need respect and compassion. Uncle Morty should picket outside *my* hospital."

We revisit the article. Morty explains:

> I'm the last guy who should be picketing. I have a brother, a sister-in-law, and two cousins who are doctors. I always get the best medical care. But what the hell is the matter with [the] people who don't [picket]? Why don't they want to do anything about it? People are so apathetic. It's unreal. They can't believe anything can be done. They think I'm a nut.

Over thirty years later, I understand Morty's frustrations. Some people *are* apathetic. Some people *can't* believe anything can be done. Some people think *I'm* a nut. Unlike my uncle, however, I'm not discouraged. I love medicine and I'm saving my profession—one doctor at a time.

"Law never was a beautiful profession for me," Morty tells the reporter. "The only aspect that ever interested me was consumer protection. The problem with law is that it only deals with money. But you take medicine—that's different, really beautiful, because it deals with people."

I turn to Mary Joy. "We don't need to picket. I don't believe in demonizing insurance or pharmaceutical companies, doctors or the AMA. Being a happy doctor is revolutionary."

"And it's catching on!" says Mary Joy.

"It is! Anyone can be a revolutionary just by being happy."

# 23

# Anti-Depressed

It's Friday night when Christie calls for an antidepressant.

I pick up on the second ring. "Hello, how can I help you?"

"This is the doctor? It's almost midnight and you answered the phone!" Frazzled, Christie tries to explain herself. "Things are kind of tough right now, Pamela. I was just calling so you could prescribe me some antidepressants."

We talk about her mother's death and the challenges of raising her autistic child.

"Christie, I'm happy to see you Saturday morning."

"I just can't believe you answered the phone. I'm so excited, I don't feel depressed anymore."

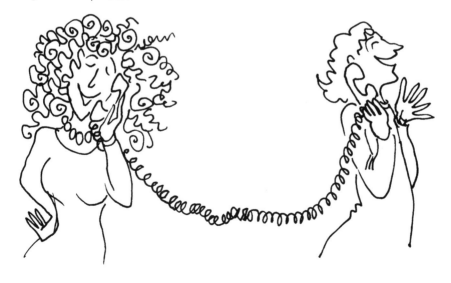

# 24

# Free Kittens

In 1997, while working for a big medical group in an industrial part of town, I arrive one morning to discover an abandoned box of kittens by the back door. I move the box into my office and tape a sign on the front of the clinic: "Free Kittens with Physical. Today Only!" Thanks to a steady stream of families in and out of my office, they all find homes by noon.

Nothing like a box of kittens to make a day at the medical mill really exciting!

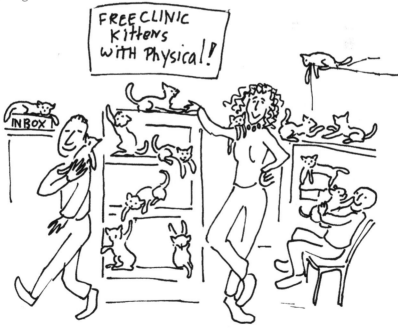

# 25

# Medical *Balderdash*

After graduating from family medicine residency, I wander around for ten years and go through a lot of jobs. During this period, my favorite employed position is at a small, doctor-owned clinic in Olympia, Washington, where I work with three older male docs and a nurse practitioner. They put me in charge of human relations. That's when the fun begins.

My colleagues let me run wild—as long as I see about thirty patients per day. I excel at the who-can-see-the-most-patients-per-day game, but prefer another kind of competition.

I start a clinic contest inspired by *Balderdash*, the board game in which players guess the definitions of unusual words. I read medical dictionaries for fun. Now I can share my dictionary addiction at work. Every Wednesday at noon, employees gather in the break room to construct definitions for obscure medical terms, while I pass out prizes. Awards go to those who create the most accurate or funniest definitions.

*Eurotophobia* is defined as the fear of female genitalia. Interestingly, the treatment is repeated exposure to naked women. Not a laughing matter for fearful patients. The funniest definition: fear of traveling with your in-laws to Europe.

*Vicarious menstruation* is actually bleeding from a surface other than the mucous membranes of the uterine cavity at the time when normal menstruation takes place. In other words, a woman gets her period, but blood doesn't drip out of her vagina. Instead, maybe it oozes from her belly button. The funniest made-up definition: getting your best friend to agree to have your period for you.

*Menhidrosis* is a form of vicarious menstruation in which a woman excretes her monthly flow through her sweat glands. Now we can diagnose the patient who walks in on a hot summer day oozing blood. The funniest definition: men who become dehydrated from sexual overexertion.

*Hircismus* is a malodorous condition of the armpits. The odor resembles that of the male goat. No kidding. That definition is straight out of a medical dictionary. The funniest definition: a hairy woman who can't stop singing Christmas songs.

*Lithopedion* is a calcified fetus trapped in a uterus. A nurse creates the funniest definition: a condition in which a woman keeps walking despite a small rock lodged inside her shoe.

*Schizotrichia* is a fancy medical term for split ends, but my colleague submits the funniest definition: a prostitute who specializes in servicing schizophrenics.

As I announce the winners, sometimes I'm laughing so hard that I pee in my pants. So I position myself next to the bathroom door. For me, it's a medical *bladder-dash*.

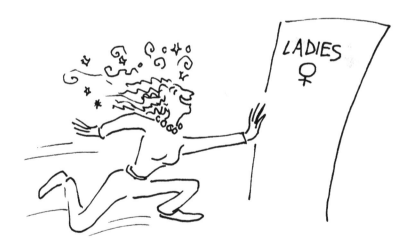

**Doctor Doin' the *Bladder-Dash***

# 26

# Pap Party

Sandra, an uninsured woman in her fifties, calls for a physical.

"When would you like to come in?" I ask.

"Well, how much is it gonna cost me, Doc?"

"Sandra, I never turn anyone away. We'll make it work. I'll do whatever you want."

"Can I bring my friend Teresa? She's uninsured and needs a physical too."

"Sure, bring all your friends!"

One week later, bursts of laughter echo down the hall as Sandra and Teresa approach. Sandra is carrying an overstuffed, brown paper sack filled with clothes.

"Hey Doc, we went through our closets, and we've got some stuff to donate if you need anything." She gives me the bag and then puts her arm around Teresa and shouts, "Woohoo! It's girls' day out!"

Teresa burps. "Excuse me, Doc. We just scarfed down an enchilada platter at the Mexican place downtown."

"Hey, we're a little tipsy from the tequila," Sandra warns. "But we're here!"

I invite them into the office and they sit together on the sofa. I pass around a tray of chocolate-covered strawberries as we review their medical histories.

Best friends for years, Sandra and Teresa have many of the same questions.

"Why do we need to keep getting Paps anyway? We had our babies.

We're done with those parts. How often do we got to get checked down there?" Teresa asks.

"Depends on what you're doing with your down-there parts," I reply.

"Doc, what's this spot on my back? It's getting bigger. Is it gonna kill me? I'm too young and beautiful to die!" Sandra exclaims.

"I've got a big mole on my butt I'd like you to check too," Teresa adds.

Their questions ring out in unison over the next ninety minutes; I do my best to keep up as I transition them into the exam room filled with balloons. I hand them each a purple flannel gown and instruct, "Everything off."

"Even our bras? And undies?" Teresa asks.

"Yep! Tell me when y'all are ready."

Moments later they shout, "We're ready!"

I discover them arm in arm on the exam table in gowns and multi-colored, knee-high striped socks. I pass each one a balloon and they pose for an impromptu photo op on my cell phone. Then I perform their physicals as they sit side by side on the exam table. First, blood pressures and pulses, and then we move head to toe and orifice to orifice. Curious, they partake in each other's exams. Taking turns in the stirrups, Teresa and Sandra even learn to perform each other's Pap smears! We're all laughing so hysterically that I feel like we're at a junior-high sleepover party.

The celebration winds down as they get dressed. At the door, I surprise them with bags of medical party favors. Sandra and Teresa each receive their own Pap smear and disposable plastic speculum in a personalized bio-hazard bag attached to a purple balloon.

Carrying on like kids at a carnival, the two promise to return next year as they skip down the hall to the lab to deposit their specimens and get their blood drawn.

I hear they did a fabulous job entertaining the phlebotomist.

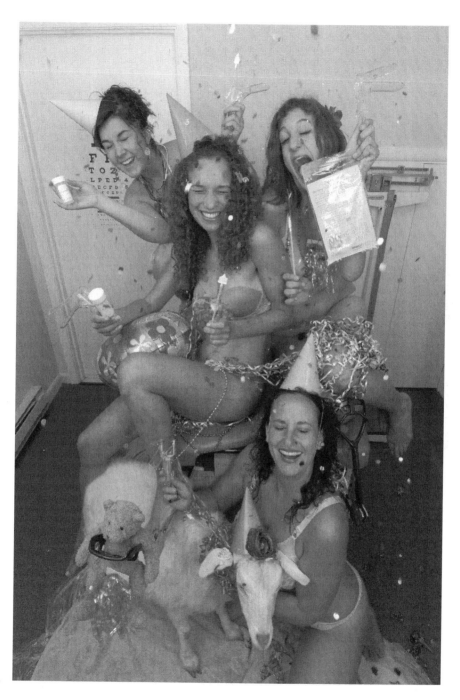

Schedule your Pap party today!

27

# A Vagina Dialogue

Sometimes pelvic exams turn into stand-up comedy. Often the doctor—unknowingly—sets up the joke. Then the patient delivers the punch line.

Today a woman in a gown awaits her pelvic exam. I approach the exam table and explain, "I need you to lie down, bend your legs, and relax your knees to the side. Then just scoot all the way down until you feel my hand."

She laughs. "You sound just like my ex-husband."

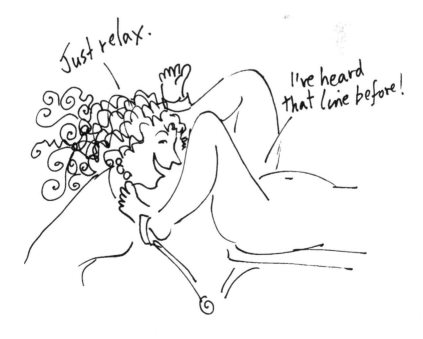

# 28

# The Laughing Vagina

Nora is a forty-year-old yoga teacher with an ovarian mass. Her mother died of ovarian cancer, so she's understandably worried. I refer her to a gynecologist. Here's what happens:

Anxiously, Nora waits in the exam room. The nurse enters and instructs, "Undress from the waist down." She hands her a paper sheet and adds, "Lie down on the table, put your feet in the stirrups, and the doctor will be right in."

The gynecologist arrives and explains, "Today, we're doing a transvaginal ultrasound. I'm applying some warm gel to the pelvic probe and now entering the vagina. What I see so far is a normal-appearing ovarian cyst."

Nora lets out a sigh of relief.

The gynecologist pauses. "So two priests and a rabbi meet in a bar on Easter . . ."

Before he finishes the joke, Nora bursts out laughing and the pelvic probe flies out of her vagina and smacks him in the face, partially dislodging his glasses and nearly knocking him off his stool.

Nora and the nurse are cracking up. The gynecologist wipes the gel from his forehead and says, "Let's try this one again. I think I set myself up and you delivered the punch line."

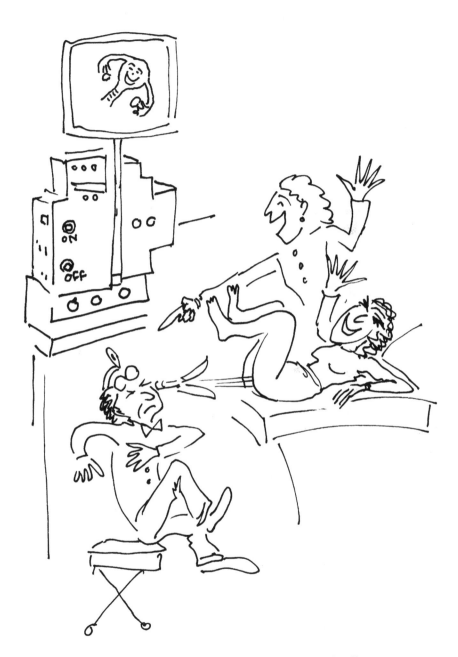

When a vagina laughs—stop, drop, and roll.

# 29

# My Favorite Phone Message

Since I have no staff or answering service, phone messages come directly to me. Patients know this, so they leave some very entertaining messages.

One woman always closes with "I love you, I love you, I love you!" and kisses into the phone, "Mwah!" Sometimes patients sing me songs. Others leave their medical complaints in poetic rhymes. This message is my all-time favorite:

> Dr. Wible! Hey, girlfriend. This is your favorite patient, Ms. Marsha—the one and only! I don't know what's going on, but there's something hanging out of my ass. I've been resting on the couch all day and it's still there. Now it's freaking me out. I'm kind of dizzy. Do you think my colon is sliding out of me and will it just keep falling all the way out? Should I push it back in with something? Maybe you have a special medical dildo for patients like me? Do you think it could be cancer? I'm not sure how to drive into town to see you with all my intestines hanging out of me, because I think I might faint. I'm getting scared out here in the woods. I was just hoping—before you become rich and famous and move out of town—that you could please just come over here and look up my ass.

Her problem? A hemorrhoid.

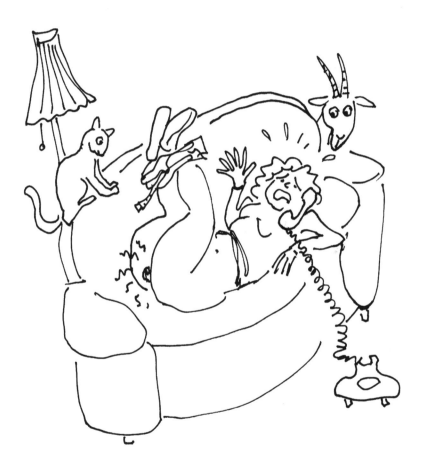

Marsha spills her guts.

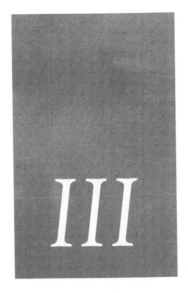

# On Creativity

Medicine is an art, but not every doctor
dreams of painting a mixed-media canvas
with a palette of earwax, baby spit,
and menstrual blood.

# 30

# Alice-in-Wonderland Medicine

Some doctors accuse me of practicing "Alice-in-Wonderland" medicine. Others believe I live in "La-La Land" or on "Planet Oregon." People have been making fun of me my entire life for being idealistic, so I'm used to it. But when our community clinic is ridiculed, I have to wonder: Why? Who could be against a community creating an ideal clinic?

While some medical journals praise our innovative model, others reject ideal care. One editor responds: "It's too utopian." Really? Can a clinic be too utopian?

I believe Americans are ready for ideal medical care. So why the resistance?

Robert F. Kennedy remarked: "One-fifth of the people are against everything all the time." I want to know why.

In 2007, I'm crisscrossing the country to recruit naysayers, after *Physicians Practice*, America's top practice management journal, invites me on a seven-city speaking tour to inspire disheartened doctors. My medical keynotes are declared "gospel revivals" by docs who envelop the stage and line the hallway, where I answer questions for hours.

Not all docs are thrilled. On stage at the Houston Convention Center, I proclaim: "Doctors deserve to be happy!" Right then, three old white guys grab their bulging bags of pharmaceutical freebies and rush out of the room.

Why resist happiness? Why oppose ideal medical care? To learn what physicians are really thinking, I review hundreds of comment cards:

She's a nut. Too ideal. Excellent and extremely informative. Complete waste of time. Thoroughly enjoyed her talk and will start a similar practice. Charming, sweet, encouraging, and completely impractical. Insightful, realistic, and quite revealing about human nature. Refreshing, but not for everyone. Excellent and so simple. Totally unreal. A bit odd. Positive, energizing, and makes you think about life/career/dreams.

And, my *favorite* comment from a physician is "Oh my! Love and peace! No help at all with reality."

Wow! Really? The fact is: patients come to us for love, peace, hope, and healing. Get it? That's the reality!

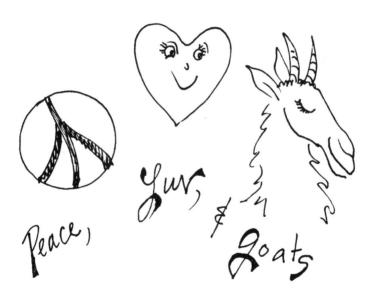

# 31

# Factory-Farmed Physicians

I was once a factory-farmed physician. Then I escaped and invited patients to design an ideal clinic. Now physicians nationwide are doing the same, leaving their jobs to create more ideal, patient-centered practices.

Maybe the term factory-farmed is too strong. Then from what precisely did we escape? To find out, I invited hundreds of free-range physicians to participate in an "antonym contest." What's the reverse of patient-centered care? What's the opposite of an ideal clinic? Here's what docs who got away report they'll never try again:

Assembly-Line Medicine
Production-Driven Health Care
McMedicine
Doc-in-a-Box
Meat-Market Medicine
Drive-By Office Visits
Take a Number
Cattle-Car Clinic
Medi-Quickie
ZombieCare
Revolving Door Practice
Freeze-Dried Med
One Size Fits None
Insti-Med
Here's-Some-Meds-Now-Get-Out Medicine

Premature Consultation
Treadmill Medicine
Rat-Race Medicine
Boot-Camp Medicine
Primarily-Don't-Care Provider
The Doctor-Patient Unrelationship
Please-Stand-Behind-Our-Bottom-Line Clinic
Shrink-Wrapped Care
What Drive$ Our Care?
We Provide: You Survive
Hamster-Wheel Medicine

And the winner? Fifty bucks goes to a physician in Florida for "Treadmill Medicine." A big thank you to all docs who are demonstrating how to get off the treadmill and care for our patients—and ourselves.

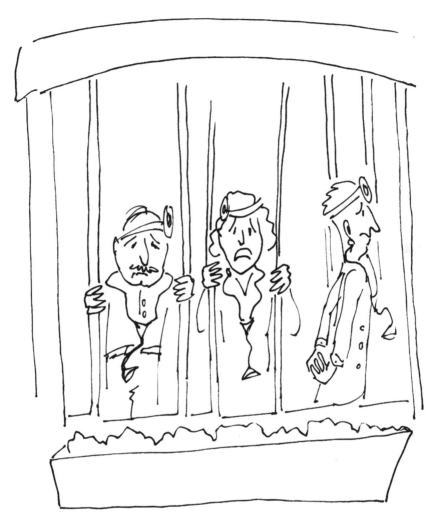

Ol' McMedicine had a farm,
Set me free! I go!
An' on that farm he had some docs,
Why? We do not know,
With a doc-doc here, and a doc-doc there,
Here a doc, there a doc, everywhere a doc-doc . . .

# 32

# What Color Is Your Diarrhea?

Medical school is white coats and white-walled hospitals—sterile, confining, and colorless. But patients are naturally colorful. I yearn to paint the stories of their lives and share them with the world.

Late one evening, I take a study break from *Harrison's Principles of Internal Medicine* and head to the closet for my art supplies. Ah, my tattered childhood box of 64 crayons—the one with the cool, built-in sharpener.

I dump them on my desk and sort through them for all skin pigments and shades of hair, for every color excreted or secreted by the human body: breast milk and earwax, menstrual blood and pus, everything from baby spit to post-nasal drip. I organize the colors on a pocket-sized chart that I laminate and carry with me on rounds. Now, curious colleagues ask to borrow my colorful card.

It's during my pediatric rotation that I realize it's no easy feat to describe the color of snot, even in my native tongue. But inevitably, on hospital rounds, a Spanish-speaking mother desperately tries to describe her infant's diarrhea. In unison, the medical team turns to me.

My attending physician looks at me lovingly, and then slowly—in a commanding voice—says, "May we please have Dr. Wible's Diarrhea Card?"

From my white-coat pocket, I retrieve my chart to display the mosaic colors of life and death: Burnt-Sienna diarrhea with a streak of Chestnut; Chartreuse sputum with clumps of Sea-Green slime; deep Mahogany clots with a splash of Torch-Red blood; Periwinkle lips and Cadet-Blue death.

As the young mother calms her firstborn at the breast, I ask, "*Señora, que color es la diarrea?*"

She points to Dandelion and Goldenrod—normal stool color for the breastfed infant.

Then comes our collective sigh of relief.

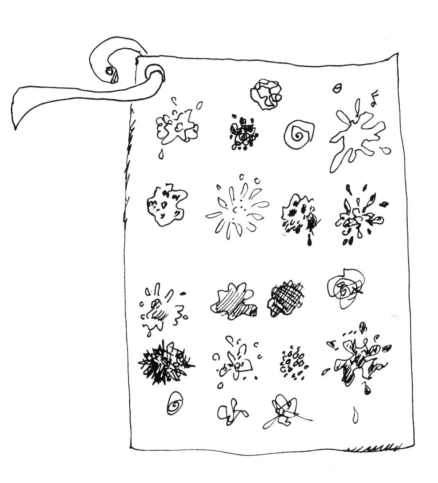

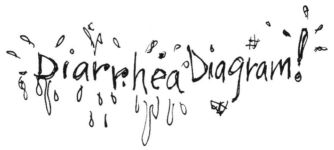

# 33

# Godiva Gallstones

On birthdays and holidays, many girls get chocolates or flowers from their fathers, but my dad is a little different.

One day I receive a package of Godiva gallstones. Wow! I imagine glistening gallbladder sacs sliced open, oozing with coconut cream, cherry chunks, or nutty nougat, and then I lift the cover off the gorgeous gold box to discover seventeen clear containers with tight-fitting lids. Arranged artfully inside—like specialty chocolates—each tiny jar a surprise: from purple-pigmented pebbles to tan tapioca pearls, tricolor treasures to jaundice-yellow gems. One has a solitary three-centimeter rock. Ouch!

An inflamed gallbladder is painful. But who gets gallstones? In medical school, they taught us a simple way to identify the typical patient. Just remember the four Fs: Fat, Fertile, Females, in their Forties. Now I'm excited every time I see heavy middle-aged women walk into the clinic.

I smile as a big lady named Belinda walks in. She says, "I got shooting pains in my belly going to my right shoulder blade, Doc."

On her exam I note pain in the right upper quadrant of her abdomen. I try to hide my excitement. "I bet you have gallstones. Let's get an ultrasound to confirm the diagnosis."

"Really? Gallstones?" she asks.

"Wait, wait, wait. I have to show you something." I open my gold box. "Look Belinda! Aren't they beautiful?"

"I got gemstones in my belly?"

"Yep!"

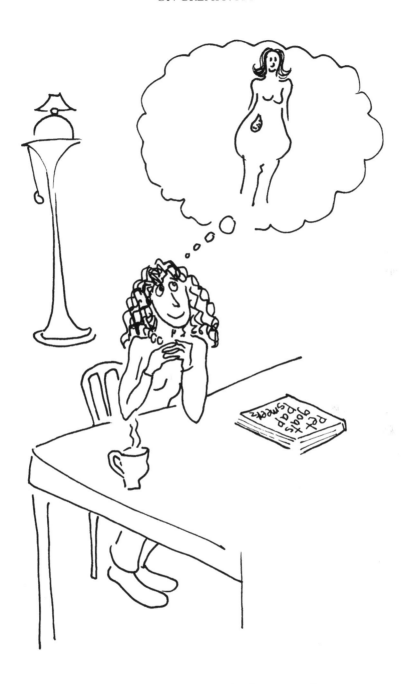

For doctors, life is a medical treasure hunt.

# 34

# Medical Waste Projects

Jennifer is here for her annual grooming. We're removing an age spot and about twenty skin tags from her neck, armpits, and groin.

"Where in the heck do all these things come from?" she asks.

"You can thank your parents, I guess."

Thirty minutes later, she's all cleaned up and ready to go when I ask, "Hey, you want to take your age spot and skin tags home?"

"Really?"

"Yep, they're inside this cute container. Makes a perfect Christmas ornament. Just dump some glitter in the preservative solution. Then add a tiny Santa statue."

"That's hilarious," Jennifer laughs. "Sure! I want to show my husband."

I properly dispose of the needle from the syringe. "Now look at this cool syringe, Jennifer. It's perfect for cleaning out earwax or dispensing liquid meds to your pets."

"I've wanted something like that for my ears."

"Wait! You're not suicidal, right?"

"No. Why?" she asks.

"Great! I have a bonus gift. How about this amazing disposable scalpel? It dices and slices and has a retractable cover and a great stainless-steel blade. Plus it comes with a built-in ruler on the handle. It only costs me $3.99, but it's yours free!"

She laughs. "You sound like you're selling kitchenware on TV! I'm sold! I'll use it for my scrapbooking project."

By the time Jennifer leaves, I've offloaded nearly all her medical waste.

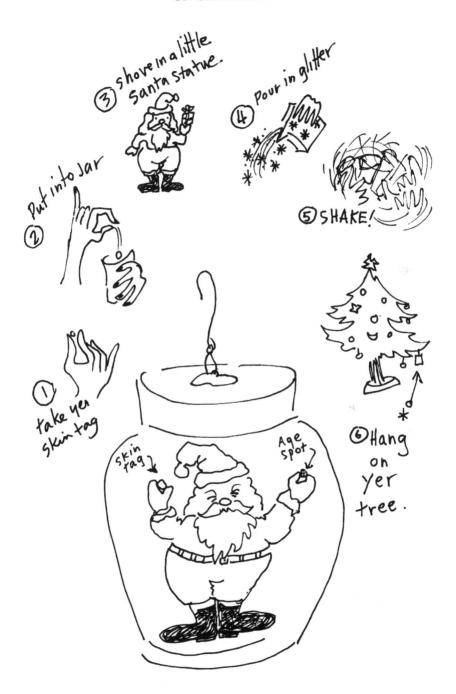

**Turning Skin Tags into Christmas Ornaments**

# 35

# Home Décor

I'm a hoarder and I'm fascinated with body parts. It's a trait inherited from Dad—a pathologist who worked as a city medical examiner.

As a child, I went to work with Dad at the morgue. In the evening I'd mill around our basement stockpiled with human remains—brains, kidneys, miscarriages, gallstones. I watched cartoons, with a human heart floating in a plastic tub atop the TV. Dad was a real pack rat.

Dad's retired now, so he passed his collection on to me. And I've passed my love of body parts on to my patients.

Don comes in today with his wife, Karen.

"I still have the growth you removed from my leg," Don boasts. "Remember, you gave it to me in a little jar? I take it out at parties and show guests when they come over. My wife prefers that I have it well hidden."

I turn to Karen. "Really? You don't like it?"

"He wants it on the shelf for display," Karen replies. "To me it's clutter. Plus it's creepy. Not everyone wants to see it."

When it comes to interior decorating, I guess not everybody has the same style.

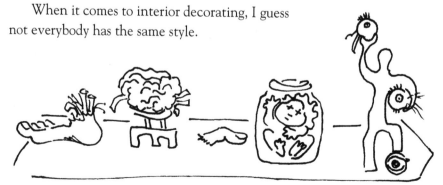

# 36

## Grow Your Greens

Yay! It's spring. Time to plant veggies.

To help patients eat garden-fresh greens, I pass out hand-decorated packages of Oregon sugar snow peas to plant in the yard. Before patients leave their appointments, I review planting instructions: put seed in ground, cover, and water—it's the easiest plant to grow. Two months later, patients share the harvest with friends and neighbors.

Sow simple. It works!

# 37

# Papping Patrice

Patrice is a forty-year-old woman who lives on a five-acre farm. She rescues animals. She lives with two goats, a sheep, a miniature donkey, an old horse, a pair of pot-bellied pigs, two barn cats, and two terriers.

Patrice hobbles in with an injured ankle. "I twisted it while chasing down the goats. I gotta get fixed up quick, Pamela. I'm going to 'The Wall' concert in two weeks with this great guy."

After examining Patrice's ankle, I reassure her and ask, "How did you meet this great guy?"

"Craigslist," she says. "He had an extra ticket to the concert and I wanted to go. We decided to meet up last weekend before the show."

"How did your first date go?"

"You'll never guess what happened! I wanted to bring my nice Coach bag, but when I opened it, there was this thing inside: plastic and papers and a little hard thing rolled up in there. I take it out and there's my missing Pap sample from last year!"

"Whoa! I was wondering why I never got your results. I thought the lab lost it. Since your Paps are always normal, I wasn't too concerned. So did you take it on your date?"

"No. I left my smear on the dresser. I thought it was gross."

"Your Pap expires after thirty days, so just throw it out. You'll need to be re-Papped, Patrice."

"But the bag says BIOHAZARD. What the heck do I do with it?" she asks.

"Bring your biohazard bag back to the clinic. Just be glad you didn't pull it out on your date! He would have thought you were a real nut job. Imagine meeting a woman online with pet goats and a Pap smear!"

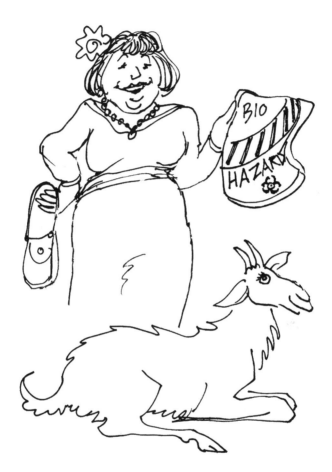

**Patrice prepares for her date.**

# 38

## A Win-Lin Situation

Lin is here for a physical. We finish early, so I entertain her by reading a few chapters I'm writing for this book.

"I love it! I wish I had more time to read."

On her way out, Lin tells me her husband is upset that I don't accept his new insurance. "Carl won't see the new doctor you suggested. He refuses to see anyone else except you. We just don't have the money to pay out of pocket."

"Don't worry. We'll figure something out. I offer a thirty percent discount if you pay at time of service. Wait, can you do editing?"

"I've edited advertising copy for thirty years. Anytime anyone has anything they're sending to a lot of people, they call me."

"That's great!"

"I even proofread the newspaper while I'm reading it every morning. When my son was little, I read his bedtime stories with a pencil in hand."

"You found mistakes in his books?"

"Yep."

"Wonderful! You help edit my book, and I'll take care of Carl."

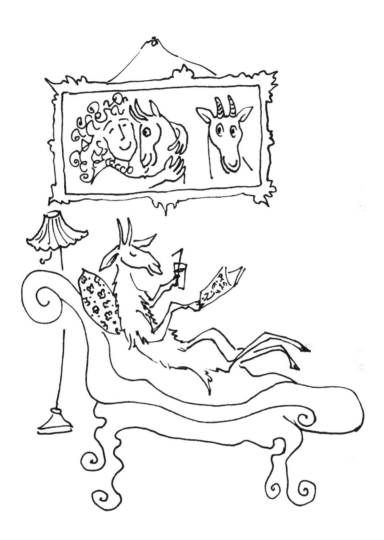

# 39

# How Fabulous!

"What would make going to the doctor fabulous?" I ask strangers as I roam around the United States with my tape recorder. From department stores to gas stations, doctors' offices to bus stops, here's how people describe fabulous health care:

The doctor's hands are always warm.

Bubble-gum-flavored medicine, lollipops, and colorful rooms.

Mutual exchange, not me complaining and the doctor fixing it.

Someone to massage my feet while waiting.

Even though I'm poor, I'd be treated like I'm rich.

No bureaucracy involved.

Getting seen within five to ten minutes.

Learning new things and enjoying the energetic rapport.

Sitting down one-on-one and not feeling like I'm rushed out.

Having an intellectual discussion with my doctor.

Hot tubs, nice couches, nice doctors.

If I wouldn't have to go into debt for health care.

Pets hanging out in the clinic.

Doctors caring about health care instead of caring about money.

Visits are thirty minutes—minimum.

No health care dependency. Health care is within you.

Receiving a yummy drink in a casual café.

If my doctor could leave her big group and do what she wants.

Friendship. The doctor is like a friend who knows me.

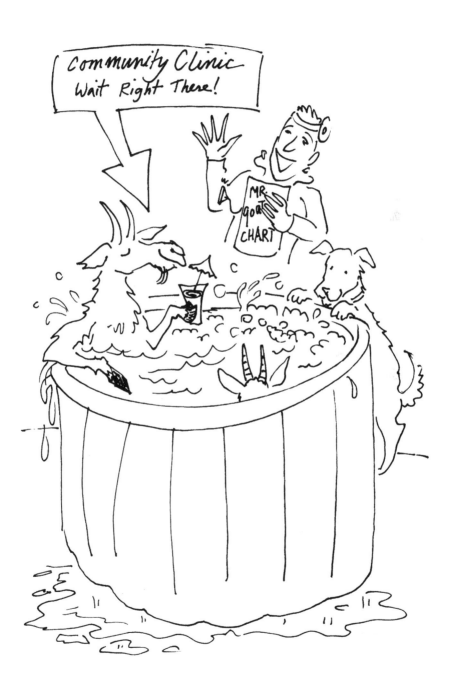

# 40

# Quit Your Job!

Amanda is a twenty-five-year-old speech therapist at a nursing home. She's back with the same complaint. "My heart is racing up to 125 beats per minute at work."

"Your labs and EKG are normal," I explain. "Avoid caffeine and stress." As she leaves I whisper, "Maybe get a different job."

A few weeks later, Amanda returns. "I'm off coffee, but my symptoms are the same."

I reply, "I'm ordering a portable device to monitor the electrical activity of your heart over the next forty-eight hours. Come back Friday for results."

Amanda is back.

"Your heart rate is high during the day," I explain, "but normal in the evenings. What do you suspect is going on?"

"I work fifty hours a week."

As she's leaving I ask, "Have you thought about quitting your job?"

I review her case with a cardiologist. He suggests a cardiac ultrasound to make sure we're not missing anything.

Amanda is back in the clinic awaiting results.

"Everything is normal, Amanda."

"But I'm doing yoga and meditation and my heart is still racing. What else can I do?"

I write her a prescription: "Quit your job."

Two weeks later, her heart rate is seventy.

"What happened?" I ask.

"I followed your prescription: I quit my job."

"It works nearly every time, for all sorts of problems—anxiety, panic attacks, depression, suicidal thoughts, fibromyalgia, carpal tunnel syndrome, high blood pressure, headaches, low sex drive, restless leg syndrome, insomnia, marital distress, neck pain, hair loss, irritable bowel syndrome, and fatigue—all with the same prescription: Quit your job."

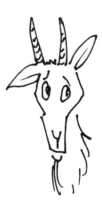

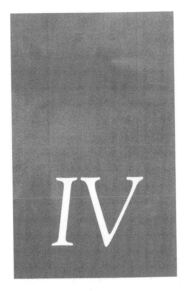

# On Compassion

Compassion means to suffer with.
I love doctoring because I'm distracted from my own pain
as I vicariously suffer with my patients. I attempt—
without judgment—to dive deep into the tragedies of
their lives and to linger there for as long as possible.
There is no billing code for compassion.
But it doesn't matter.
Insurance companies never pay for pain and suffering,
but the wisdom I have gained is priceless.

# 41

# Bambi Syndrome

Life changes in a heartbeat.

In the "Events of the Cardiac Cycle" lab, four students are assigned to each dog. Instructions:

> Inject the live dog with epinephrine and study the EKG. Sever cardiac nerves. Carve open the chest and shock the heart. As the dog's blood pressure drops, remove the heart. Now, stab the aorta with a scissor blade and slice open the ventricle. Check for heartworms. Bag the carcass, and clean your instruments and work station.

To be a healer, I'm being forced to kill. But murder is not part of my curriculum. So I sign the papers to drop out of medical school. But I can't leave. With an apartment full of pets, no money for a U-Haul, and no clear destination, I'm unable to garner sympathy—even from my parents. My anatomy partner advises, "Just keep taking tests until you figure out what you want to do."

At age twenty-two, I decide to fight for my life. In a petition, I state my personal intention not to kill, and circulate the petition to classmates. From among the 189 students, three share my moral objections and sign on. I circulate a second petition for others to support our right to opt out of animal labs, but no classmates sign due to "fear of being blacklisted from residencies."

Then I send a letter to the physiology director stating that "I will not participate in animal experiments."

"These are not animal experiments," he responds. "They are *experiences*. Attendance is mandatory. You are assigned to Team 11B. An unexcused absence will compromise your teammates' education and prevent your matriculation into the clinical core."

So I forward my petition to the dean of medicine, who requires that I meet with him. I enter his office and sit in a large mahogany chair across from the sixty-year-old physician.

I begin with a personal statement of my values and priorities: "I am vegan. I do not eat or wear animal products. I am morally opposed to injuring animals and will not participate in these labs."

He stares at me quizzically. Then—with an authoritarian, yet paternal, even loving tone—he diagnoses me with "Bambi Syndrome" and grants my exemption. I'm relieved that I will not have to kill a dog to become a doctor.

My relief is short-lived. The next week, while studying, I see a cart full of dogs wagging their tails. As they pass by my classroom, I panic. My vision narrows and blurs. My heart is racing and I feel like I'm going to faint.

An hour later, classmates emerge splattered with blood. Men boast of their conquests. Bags overflow with carcasses—man's best friend slaughtered in cold blood.

Walking home, I'm crying not only for the loss of our innocent, ever-faithful friends, but also for my classmates, methodically dehumanized right in front of me.

I cry myself to sleep holding my dog, Happy. The next morning, it's impossible to return to class. With swollen eyelids, completely sealed shut, I can no longer bear to see the brutality.

Nearing graduation, we're all so excited. While completing residency applications, fellow classmates beg me to write their personal statements for them.

"But a personal statement is personal," I say. "How could I possibly write *your* personal statement?" In the end, my classmates are blacklisted, not from their residencies, but from their own identities. Medical education too often robs us of our souls, ourselves—our very humanity.

Bambi Syndrome saved my life. I've never been so happy to be diagnosed with a disease.

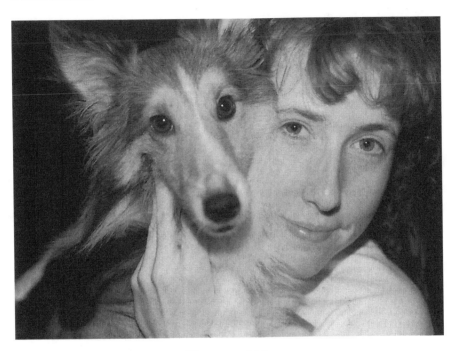

**Happy and Me**

# 42

# Acute Liberal Delusion

April 1992. University of Texas Medical Branch at Galveston. I'm a third-year medical student working on the psychiatric unit. I'm searching for my patient's chart when I discover *mine* . . . labeled with my misspelled name and presumed diagnosis: Wibel, Pam, Room 140A, Acute Liberal Delusion.

I open the chart. It's empty. I'm an easy target: I'm the only woman on a team of male medical students—good old boys passing through on their way to surgery and radiology (lucrative specialties). I reflect on our recent conversations on the psychiatric unit.

The guys on my team frequently say, "Pam, you're a flower child from the '60s."

(These are among the same guys who will ask me to write their personal statements for their residency applications.)

I smile. "Thanks. You never met a flower child?"

They tell me I'm their first.

"I never met any good old boys. Y'all think it's fun to get drunk, play golf, and go hunting, right? That's pretty weird."

"That's normal around here, Pam. That's what people do."

Before medical school, I spent four years at Wellesley College with progressive women, so meeting these guys is a real treat. I listen to their stories and find them oddly fascinating. I'm sure the intrigue is mutual.

With equal curiosity, I listen to my patients' stories. But in medicine, listening is undervalued; and in psychiatry, the fastest way out of the room is to diagnose and drug. Once patients are labeled, there's no reason to chit-chat. Why sit in a room with a schizophrenic when you could be on the golf course drinking beer with your buddies?

But I learn a lot listening to my psych patients. Reviewing their charts, I discover patients' diagnoses change with each admission. Sometimes, the same patient can be bipolar, then paranoid schizophrenic, and then depressed and suicidal. Why? When I listen long enough, they confide: "Doctors are the crazy ones."

It's hilarious that psychiatric patients believe psychiatrists need psychiatric help, but most docs I know seem emotionally unbalanced—myself included—so I can't disagree. I've been studying doctors my entire life. Physicians are seriously restrained and guarded—compared to artists and musicians.

Some of the greatest artists and writers were mentally ill. In fact, there's a link between mental illness and genius. Vincent van Gogh was bipolar. Ernest Hemingway and Abraham Lincoln were severely depressed and suicidal. With enough sleep deprivation we all start hallucinating. I'm thinking I'd rather hang out with van Gogh while he's hallucinating than get drunk and go hunting with my classmates.

Listening with an open heart and mind is an act of courage. I peel the label off my chart and glue it into my diary under the heading: "Medicine's attempt to destroy my inherent compassion and loving spirit."

WIBEL, PAM 140-A

Dx: ACUTE LIBERAL DELUSION

CAT. NO. CL- 1

# 43

# Alternative Medicine

I'm passing through the frozen foods department at the grocery store when I run into a local physician.

"So how's your new clinic going?" he asks.

"I'm loving it. I'm spending thirty to sixty minutes with each patient."

"You actually spend time with patients? That's *very* alternative."

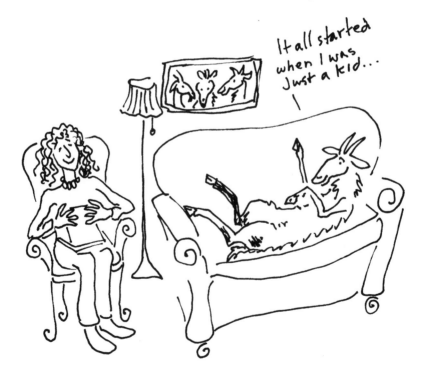

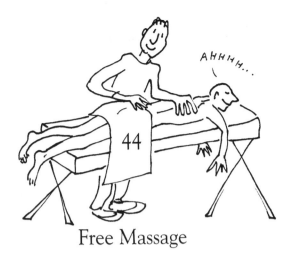

## Free Massage

One afternoon, I hire a patient—a massage therapy student—to work on low-income, high-needs psychiatric clients during their medical appointments. All enjoy free footbaths and hand rubs. Not one had ever received massage; most had never experienced safe, loving touch in their lives. Now they require less medication.

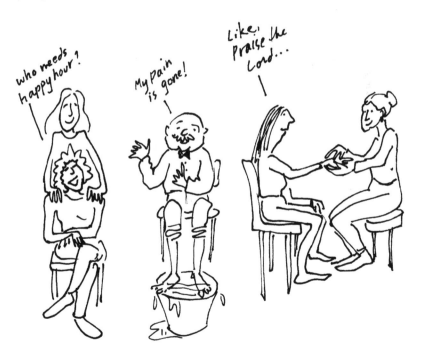

**A waiting room morphs into a medical massage parlor.**

# 45

# Medical Marijuana

Jesse and Tanya came to see me for the first time six months ago. Jesse worked for nine years as an organic produce distributor, but he's unemployed now. Tanya is completing her music degree at the university. They're uninsured and need a doctor. Both have skin problems and Jesse has chronic neck pain. He has used medical marijuana for years to cope with the pain.

Today Jesse is back. "I'm coughing up yellow mucous and wheezing real bad at night."

I examine him and prescribe antibiotics for pneumonia. "So how's everything else going?"

"Not great. I'll be doing three years in Idaho for marijuana possession."

"What happened?"

"My ex-stepmom is in Idaho, where she's getting radiation for a tumor in her nose. It's the size of a lemon and it's distorting her face. She's in a ton of pain. She said she'd benefit from medical marijuana, but it's not prescribed there."

"So you brought her some marijuana?"

"Well, I didn't think it through too well. I'm not gonna lie, Doc. I did need the extra cash. I figured I'd take enough to supply anyone in need."

"You took a supply for the entire state of Idaho? How much did you take?"

"Three duffle bags. They value it at $150,000."

In Oregon, a medical card allows each patient six plants, eighteen seedlings, and no duffle bags.

"So how did you get caught, Jesse?"

"I got pulled over by an Oregon State Trooper for speeding."

"You were speeding with $150,000 of pot in your car?"

"He asked if I had any marijuana. I showed him a small stash and told him I didn't have my medical card with me. He called to check my record and then let me go, with a warning. I felt really lucky, but two hours later, I was pulled over in Idaho and asked if I had anything in the car. I said I had a small amount of medicine. They searched the car and found sixty-eight pounds of pot and hauled me off to the county jail."

"That sucks."

"It got bad, Doc. In jail, I told them that I don't eat dairy or meat for religious reasons. I wasn't given a vegetarian diet for eight days. When the doctor finally saw me, I'd lost a bunch of weight. I told him that the only reason I didn't lose more is that I traded food with other inmates so I could get some of their boiled cabbage and carrots. Due to my food trades, he placed me in solitary confinement. Eventually they gave me vegetarian meals, loaded with butter and cheese. He said he wanted to see if I really couldn't eat dairy. You'd think they'd feed prisoners healthy to save on health care costs. I made bail twelve days later. By then, I'd lost seventeen pounds, over ten percent of my body weight."

"That's horrible, Jesse."

"In the end, I'm doing three years behind bars because I was trying to make the world a better place."

"By trying to get medication to people who need it? You were basically on a medical mission to Idaho?"

"Yes, Doc."

"But how do you know all the pot would've gone to patients with medical needs?"

"With the black market, I couldn't guarantee that it would all end up in the hands of medical patients. I think most people who use marijuana are self-medicating in some way."

"You're probably right, Jesse." I pause to contemplate. "So how are you feeling?"

"I'm scared as hell. I'm scared of dying in prison from poor medical care, tooth decay, fights. I'm scared I'll never see my family again. We got a fifteen-year-old daughter, a freshman in high school. She's a straight-A student. I'm worried she'll get depressed and her grades will drop. I want to start my prison sentence next week so I can get out in time to see her walk down the aisle at graduation. I'm gonna miss meeting her first real boy-friend, seeing her go to prom."

"That's really sad, Jesse"

"And I'm afraid my wife won't make it financially. I'm afraid she'll get lonely, find another man. We've been married fourteen years, together sixteen. It's a fear that's building up in me, Doc."

"What are you doing to prepare for all of this?"

"We gotta move out of our rental. It's too expensive. Then I gotta get my wife and daughter into low-income housing. But my wife will have to sign a document that I can't live there."

"Why?"

"I'm a documented felon."

"What's upsetting you most?" I ask.

"Every time I watch the news and hear about violent criminals—rapists, kidnappers, child molesters—sent to prison for less time than me, I feel sick."

"Maybe you can get out early."

"With marijuana it's mandatory minimum, no early release."

"Anything else I can do for you today, Jesse?"

"I got a mole on my chest. I noticed it two weeks ago."

I examine his mole. "It looks a little suspicious. Ordinarily, I'd keep an eye on it, but if I'm not going to see you for three years, we better remove it before you go to prison. After everything you've been through, I'm not gonna let a melanoma take you down."

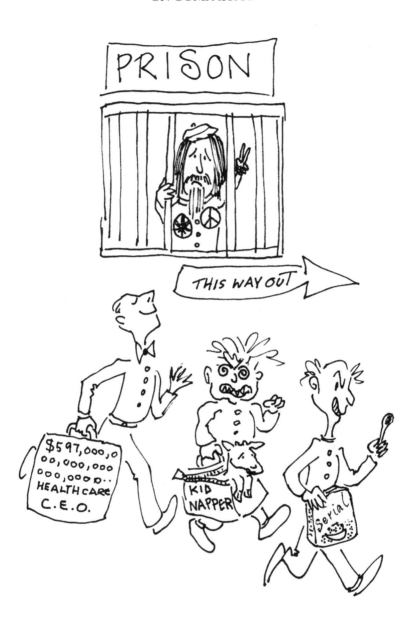

# 46

# Fukushima Colonoscopy

Tom is an uninsured sixty-year-old man with irritable bowel syndrome. For years I've been recommending he get a screening colonoscopy.

"So, Tom, where ya at on the colonoscopy?"

"I'm not looking forward to having a guy shove a tube up my butt, and I don't have an extra two or three grand just sitting around, ya know."

It's not easy convincing Tom to sign up, but he finally agrees to get one this year.

"Tom, the prep is the worst part: a liquid diet, laxatives, and lots and lots of bowel movements. You'll need to spend twenty-four hours near the toilet."

"I've got irritable bowels. I stay close to toilets, Doc. I'll let you know how it goes."

After the procedure, Tom facebooks me to share his experience:

> Doc, the worst part of my procedure wasn't the procedure or the prep. The worst part of my procedure was in the waiting room, staring at a fifty-inch flat-screen TV with CNN talking about the nuclear disaster. A waiting room should be a quiet place to contemplate or read. The last thing a patient needs to listen to is Fox News anchor propaganda or CNN's breaking news of the latest tragedy. If health care is about caring, then why scare the shit out of people in the waiting room?

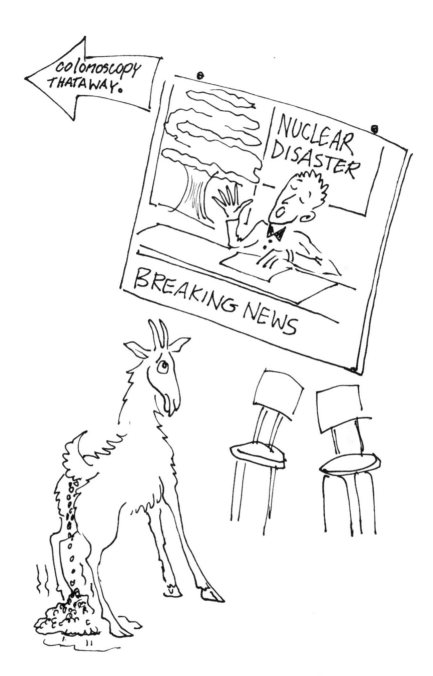

A Pre-Apocalyptic Colonoscopy Prep

# 47

# Adult Diapers

Ken is a sixty-two-year-old postal worker who has been suffering with diarrhea for fifteen years.

"So how did the diarrhea start?" I ask.

"I was lonely and depressed. I ate an entire bag of candy when nobody came to the door for Halloween. After that, I was unable to keep food down; I lost weight. Then I had blood in my stool. The doctor did a colonoscopy and told me I had ulcerative colitis."

"How have you been lately?"

"I had one bloody stool after eating some raw lettuce a few years ago. As long as I avoid raw vegetables and stress, I don't get bloody diarrhea."

"But you still have diarrhea?"

"Yes. Doctor, I'm afraid to leave home in the morning unless I have two bowel movements. Diarrhea comes without warning. I've had accidents at work."

"How much water are you drinking?"

"I don't like water. But I know I'm supposed to drink a lot of water, so I carry a water bottle and drink sips constantly. If I don't have my bottle, I get stressed."

"When did you start drinking so much water, Ken?"

"I had a snoring condition and a dry mouth years ago, so a doctor mentioned that perhaps I wasn't drinking enough water."

"How often are you urinating?"

"Twice an hour, all morning long. And if I hold my bladder too long, I get diarrhea."

I review his diet and recommend, "Stop drinking so much water. Don't drink with meals. And add a tablespoon of ground flaxseed with meals."

Two weeks later, Ken stops by before he and his wife take off for a romantic getaway to Bali.

"Are you excited about your trip?"

"Oh yes, Doctor. And the diet is working. We were considering buying adult diapers for the trip. But my diarrhea is gone!"

# 48

# I Dream of Toilets

I love this place. I graduated from residency here more than a decade ago. Now I'm invited back to the University of Arizona Department of Family and Community Medicine to teach the next generation of doctors.

Sitting in a circle with third-year residents, I feel hopeful. Some of the docs are tired, but they don't have the glazed-over, worn-out look of many doctors I meet. Just underneath their fatigue, I feel their exuberance, their excitement.

I ask residents to describe their dream clinics.

They seem surprised. One resident responds, "In three years of training, nobody has ever asked us about our dreams."

"Today, I welcome you all to imagine the clinic of your dreams. What would it look like?"

"Oh. Wow," the woman next to me responds. "I'd live with refugees from Africa in the apartments down the street and deliver their babies." Her passion is contagious.

The guy beside her begins to smile. "I'll return to my hometown," he says, "and open a sports medicine clinic in a local gym."

And the young lady across from him bursts forth with her plan. "I'd like to start an organic farm where patients come over for lunch and even get a haircut! Plus—I'll have on-site child care and yoga classes."

The doctor to her left starts to cry. "I just returned from a weeklong yoga retreat," she shares. "There, everyone was assigned a job. I cleaned the outhouses. Every day I scrubbed the toilets. And my toilets were really clean. I felt a sense of accomplishment—a level of satisfaction I never feel with patients." She pauses before revealing her truth: "I'd rather clean toilets than see patients."

I know her pain. Doctors are perfectionists, but patients are imperfect. They smoke, eat crappy food, get sick, and die. Sometimes, cleaning toilets is easier than curing patients.

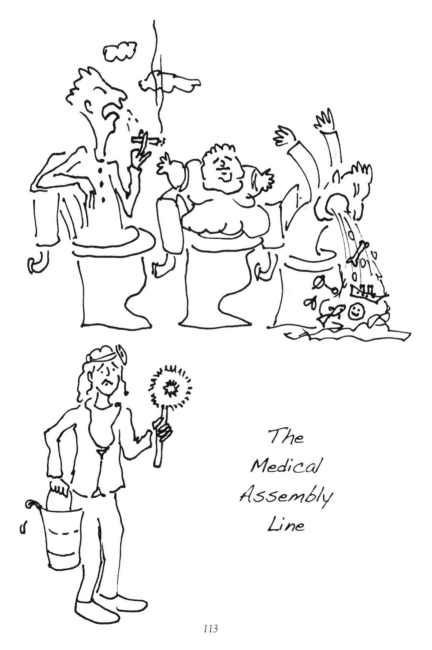

The
Medical
Assembly
Line

# 49

# A Pap Talk

Brandi is a thirty-two-year-old mother who comes in for her Pap. She arrives with her partner, her one-year-old daughter, five-year-old son, and shy eleven-year-old stepdaughter, Sarah, who sinks into the beanbag in the corner with a book.

"How long has it been since your last Pap?" I ask.

"Five years." Brandi turns to Sarah and exclaims, "Hey, Sarah! Pay attention! You're gonna need a Pap in a few years too."

"What?" I ask Brandi. "Sarah just turned eleven. She won't need a Pap until she's twenty-one or sexually active."

"Really?" asks Brandi.

"And when did you become sexually active?" I ask.

"Sixteen."

"So when did you get your first Pap?"

"Thirteen."

"You lost your virginity with your doctor?!" I exclaim.

"What?" Brandi looks at me like I'm crazy.

"Okay, let's start over. Everyone listen up." The whole family gathers around. "Brandi, do you know why you are getting a Pap?"

"To check stuff out down there?" she asks.

"What stuff?" I ask.

"To check for cancer cells."

"Of what?" I ask.

Brandi hesitates. "The cervix?"

"Yes! The Pap smear checks for cervical cancer, which is caused by a sexually transmitted infection—the human papillomavirus. So nuns and virgins don't really need Paps."

I look at Sarah. "Don't worry. You won't need a Pap until *after* you are sexually active." Then I turn back to Brandi. "Plus, I'd prefer that Sarah's first sexual experience be with someone other than me."

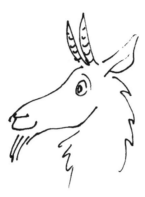

# 50

# Maria's First Pap

Maria just turned twenty-one and has a serious boyfriend. She has been sexually active for two years. She's here for her first Pap smear.

We chat for a few minutes. She seems nervous, so I introduce her to the instruments.

"This is the speculum we'll be using. It shouldn't be too uncomfortable. It's smaller than most things that have been in there. It's kind of like a vaginal shoehorn."

Maria changes into her gown and I guide her feet into the stirrups covered with pink polka-dot socks. "Just trying to keep things fun!" I laugh.

"Thanks," she says, "but let's get this over with."

"So do you know what I'm checking for on a Pap smear?"

"Not really."

"It's a screening test for cervical cancer. The Pap smear was named after this Greek doctor, George Papanicolaou. He came up with this idea one hundred years ago."

"Women have been getting Paps for a hundred years?"

"Yep! Just be glad you weren't his wife. Her name was Lady Mary Papanicolaou and she was his assistant. He needed a female volunteer, so she submitted to the first Pap smear."

"That sounds horrible!"

"Lady Mary Papanicolaou was a real trooper. She apparently submitted to a Pap every day for twenty-one years while her husband worked on the development of the Pap smear!"

"What a marriage!"

"Okay, we're done. That wasn't so bad, was it?"

"It's over? That was easy," Maria says.

"Would you like your plastic speculum as a souvenir?"

"Umm . . . that's okay. You can keep it."

"Are you sure, Maria? The speculum is a wonderful instrument to have in your home medical kit. It was even used in ancient Greece. Exams were so exciting back then that women used to line up in the streets to get in."

"I think I better watch out for Greek men. I'm not really that adventurous down there."

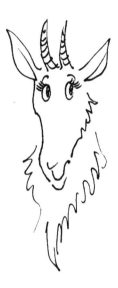

# 51

# Melissa's New Job

Melissa is a beautiful brunette in her thirties. She's honest, open-minded, intelligent, and very funny. She's been a great friend for years and we hang out socially. In fact, I was just over to her house for dinner. Today, she's here for her Pap. I ask the standard questions before her exam.

"How many sexual partners have you had in the last year?"

"I've just started a new line of work," she replies. "I'm a sex worker now. I was tired of telemarketing. I'm more of a sensual artist and healer."

"How many clients have you had?"

"Five so far. Mostly older men who have lost their wives. One younger guy was really hot. I would have dated him," she laughs.

"What's it like with the older men?"

"Some of them just want to talk. One asked if it would be okay to kiss me. They are very respectful."

"Do you feel like you are healing them?"

"Yes. I just channel my sensual energy and help them know that it's natural and healthy to be adored and indulged."

"Hmm . . . so how much do you get paid?"

"Two hundred dollars per hour."

"More than most doctors! Maybe I'll switch careers," I joke. "So any specific concerns today?"

"I'd like to know how to protect myself and my lover from diseases."

"Oh, right, your lover. What does he think of your new career?"

"He's okay with it. We just want to be safe."

"What types of sexual activities are you involved in with your clients, and do you use barrier protection?"

"I'm using condoms for vaginal and anal sex. I'm not using anything for oral sex. So how likely am I to contract gonorrhea or chlamydia from oral sex, and could I pass it on to my lover or another man?"

"Very unlikely. HIV can be transmitted orally, especially if you've had recent dental surgery. Don't brush your teeth after oral sex, because the bristles can scratch your gums and invite infection. Chew gum instead."

We discuss many other infections, and I answer her questions to the best of my ability as we complete her exam. "I'll be in touch with results," I add. "Call if you need anything."

Melissa is back to get checked for oral gonorrhea. "Hey Pamela, it's been six months since I've started my new job, and I'm having a totally wonderful experience at it."

"What's so wonderful about your job?"

Melissa looks straight into my eyes. "It's the first job I've had where people are truly grateful."

I've spent over twenty years listening to patients, and I've never heard anyone speak with such love and appreciation for their work.

"That's beautiful, Melissa." I pause to take a breath.

She continues, "I'm well paid, I get to try new things, and getting dressed up for work is super fun with mostly cute lingerie."

"Plus you're self employed! You're not working on an assembly line and you can set your own hours." I note the similarities in our work.

"How many partners do you have per month?" I ask.

"I get plenty of repeats. I have sex, including oral sex, with twenty to twenty-five people a month. Is that a huge number?"

"Umm—compared to a nun—yes."

"Oh, plus some trios with other sex workers."

"Usually two women and a man?" I ask.

"Yeah. I know it sounds like a lot of people, but nearly fifty percent never have intercourse with me and twenty-five percent have intercourse with me for two minutes or less."

"Two hundred dollars for two minutes! Why only two minutes? Oh, right, premature ejaculation and erectile dysfunction."

"Yes. So I'm not actually having a lot of sex. I'm kissing, touching, doing massage. The truth is I have more sex with my lover in one evening than I do in three months working."

"How do you figure that, Melissa?"

"My partner lasts three hours."

"Fascinating." I pause to consider the situation. "Hey, at your two-minute rate that's $18,000! That's more than a neurosurgeon."

As I swab her throat for gonorrhea, she gags.

"Sorry, Melissa. That was probably worse than a blow job."

She laughs. "It was. So, Pamela, how's your love life?"

I update Melissa on my recent adventures, and then read her a few chapters I'm working on for this book. "Hey, want to be in the book? You could be the centerfold!"

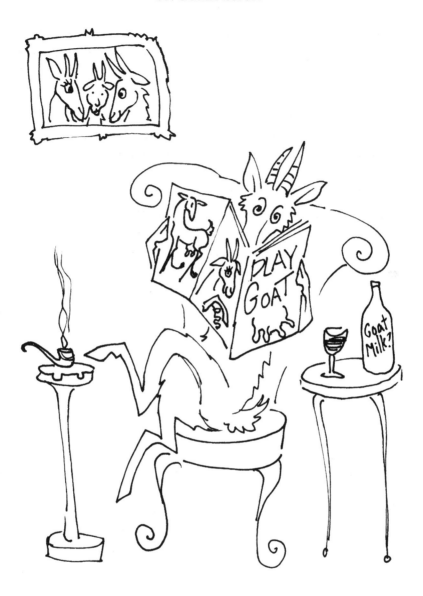

# 52

# A Tale of Two Testicles

Evan, a retired police officer, calls for an urgent appointment. I can hear the angst in his voice.

"Sure Evan, come right over."

An hour later, he arrives in obvious distress. "I gotta show you something, Doc." We proceed to the exam room. He pulls his pants down and points to his left testicle. I put on gloves, turn on the exam light, and I lean in real close.

"What's the problem?" I ask.

"Look, Doc. Can't you see?"

"What?"

"My left testicle is hanging real low."

"That's it? No pain?"

"No pain. But look how low it is!"

I stand up. "Evan, here's the deal: most people hang lower on the left. In women, the left breast is slightly larger and hangs lower. For men, the left testicle generally hangs lower. So you're in with the main crowd."

"I've been this way my entire life?"

"Yep. You're normal."

Evan smiles. Relieved, he hands me his co-pay and a five-dollar tip. As he leaves, I add, "Just so ya know, most curvy penises also curve to the left."

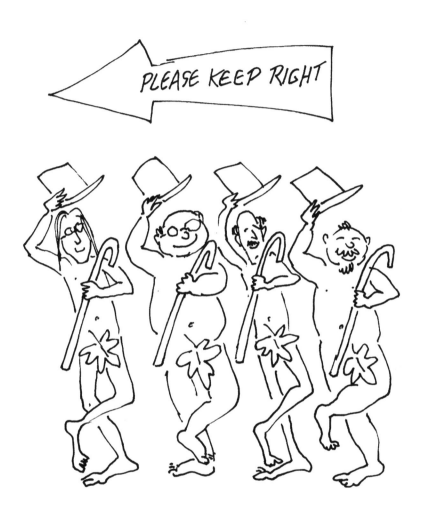

Most men lean to the left.

# 53

# Gown Etiquette

In our community clinic, paper gowns are out. Cloth gowns are in. The purple flannel gowns are my favorite. They were handmade by a patient in exchange for medical care.

Before physicals, I place a periwinkle, terry-cloth drape over the exam table. On top of the drape is a neatly folded flannel gown. Finally, atop the gown, I place a single dark-chocolate heart covered in pink foil. It's like the truffle on your pillow at upscale hotels.

John, a fifty-year-old man, is here for his physical. Accompanying me is Susie, a twenty-year-old premedical student at the local university. I tell John, "This is Susie, a student working with me today. Do you mind if she sits in on your visit?"

"No problem. The more the merrier!" he replies.

Entering the exam room, John lifts the gown off the exam table and asks a common question: "How do you put this thing on? Does it open to the front or the back?"

"There is no perfect way to wear a gown," I explain, "because I need to see everything. The best gown is no gown at all."

Susie and I step out of the room. "Let us know when you're ready," I yell back at John, and then I tell Susie, "It's weird. Women always want gowns. But pretty much all men have their physicals in the buff."

"I'm ready!" says John, and we enter the room. He's sitting naked on the table. As I'm taking his blood pressure and pulse, Susie is standing in front of him, almost directly over him. I attempt to signal her to the side without success.

"Wow," John jokes, "I've got two beautiful women. It's a two-for-one."

His blood pressure and heart rate are usually normal, but now both are really high. I think to myself: his blood pressure and heart rate are elevated because an attractive twenty-year-old woman is standing directly in front of a naked fifty-year-old man. It's biological.

The rest of his exam is normal. I'm just glad he didn't get an erection.

"John, your blood pressure and heart rate are high, but I'm not holding it against you."

Here's what I learned today about gown etiquette. Fifty-year-old men should *gown-up* when in the presence of twenty-year-old women.

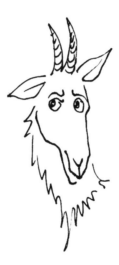

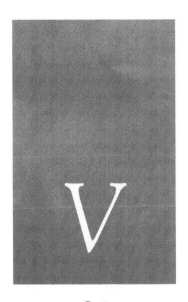

V

# On Teaching

*If doctors are victims, patients learn to be victims.*
*If doctors are discouraged, patients learn to be discouraged.*
*If we want happy, healthy patients, why not start*
*by filling our clinics with happy, healthy doctors?*

# 54

# Doctor-in-Training—Part One

Both my parents are physicians. They are never home much because they work all the time. With no reliable child care, Dad takes me to work. The morgue is my favorite spot. It's like our secret clubhouse. Nobody ever bothers us there.

Entering the morgue, Dad opens the stainless-steel doors to the cooler and says, "Good morning! Is anyone home?" Then Dad props me up and introduces me to everyone. Today he announces, "Look! It's Sally!"

I interview Sally while Dad examines body parts in a bucket by the sink. I always have a lot to talk about. I tell Sally all about my life and ask all about her life too. Leading with an open-ended question, I ask, "So how are things going for you?" I pause. Then I answer for her. I assume Sally is a brave woman who has led a heroic life. Dad says she's probably a single mom, her life cut short by poverty. He eventually goes along with my version.

Dad and I work lots of odd jobs. Though his main job is at the hospital, Dad takes random jobs for the city, where he helps even more people in medical crisis. Leaving the morgue, we head to the drug addiction clinic and then work the night shift at the police station.

At the addiction clinic, in Camden, New Jersey, I sit between Dad and his clients. Dad introduces me the same way every time. "This is Pamela. She's a doctor-in-training. Show her your track marks."

Today it's Mr. Jones who rolls up his sleeves to display his scarred arms. After a brief exam, Dad—a philosophy major in college—offers this guy all sorts of advice.

"How many kids do you have?" Dad begins.

"Got three, Doc. Twin girls and a boy."

"How much money do you estimate that you have spent on heroin in the last ten years?"

"Not sure, Doc."

Dad does a few calculations on a scrap of paper. He shows Mr. Jones the total. "With the money you spent on heroin, you could have sent all your kids to a fine community college and had enough left over for a car."

"Probably right."

Dad looks at Mr. Jones and admits, "I got an addiction too," as he pulls out a bag of banana-flavored Circus Peanut marshmallow candies. "I love Circus Peanuts, but I've had this unopened bag in my desk for two years. I don't allow my addiction to control me."

As Mr. Jones stands up to leave, Dad asks, "Do you have any words of wisdom for our doctor-in-training?"

"Don't do drugs," says Mr. Jones. "Save your money. Your dad is a very smart man."

At noon, Dad passes out lunch money to clients in need. He hands ten bucks to a transsexual woman in a head wrap and tells us to "go have fun." So I spend the afternoon on a street corner with recovering heroin addicts, eating pizza and learning Puerto Rican Spanish slang from a sexy black woman with huge biceps.

Then we head to the Philadelphia jail, where we evaluate drunk drivers. Every eighth night, Dad and I have a slumber party at the police station. We set up our cots in a cinder-block room with Dad's name on the door. Every week, I'm given a new policeman coloring book with a fresh box of crayons. Coloring the same policeman on horseback each week bores me, so I get clearance to interview the inmates.

"Don't get close to the bars or they'll grab you," the guard warns. But I'm never afraid.

In the first cell are three cackling black women. In the next, an old, naked white lady masturbates against the bars. I sit down in front of a caged, middle-aged white woman. She says, "Hey kid, get me a cigarette."

"Why?"

"Helps me cope."

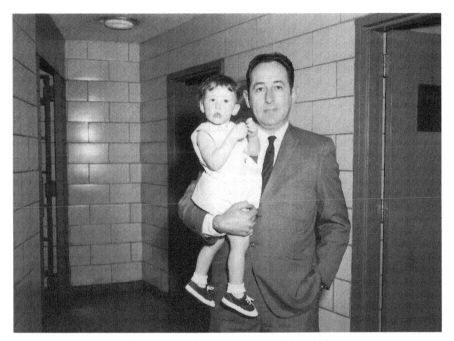

**Me and my dad work the night shift.**

"Okay, I'll check." I tell the guard, "That lady over there wants a smoke." Then I wander off with Dad down the hall.

At midnight, Dad and I are sleeping when suddenly there's a *Bang! Bang! Bang!* on our door. The policeman says, "Hey, Doc, we got some 1037s (a code number for a DUI)."

"Okay. How many do you have?" Dad asks.

"We got three waiting for you."

"Let's bring them in one at a time." Dad moves to his desk as a black man staggers into our room and sits in a folding metal chair across from Dad.

"Mr. Johnson, I'm the police doctor and this is Pamela, a doctor-in-training. I'd like to ask you a few questions. Have you been drinking?"

"Huh? Uh . . . yeah."

"What were you drinking?"

"Jus' a nip of Thunderbird."

"I'd like you to do several tests for me. Lean forward and breathe toward me." Dad notes the smell of alcohol. Then he has Mr. Johnson do the walk-the-line test. But Mr. Johnson stumbles and leans against the wall. Dad types up a few things on his manual typewriter and Mr. Johnson leaves, just as the next man staggers in.

We talk to drunk men all night. On an average Christmas Eve, we see up to thirty prisoners during our twelve-hour shift, but if there's a big snowstorm we might only get eight. Dad estimates he has seen 13,500 DUIs over all the years he has worked there.

We also spend two nights each month at the state psychiatric hospital talking to schizophrenics. Plus we're on call for the Philadelphia Fire Department twice per month. Sometimes we get calls to go to huge apartment fires at two o'clock in the morning. I usually sit in the lead fire truck and drink hot chocolate while talking with the crew.

I learn to interview patients by watching Dad. He introduces me the same way to every patient: "This is Pamela. She's a doctor-in-training. Do you mind if she sits here while I talk to you?" Nobody ever says no.

After work, we return to our suburban neighborhood where I find my friends playing house with dolls. My best friend keeps begging me to play. But playing house is never my thing. And playing with Barbies just seems silly after examining real people.

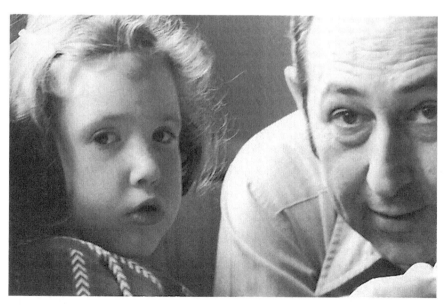

**Me and Dad**

# 55

## Doctor-in-Training—Part Two

I've been practicing medicine nearly twenty years, but I'm still a doctor-in-training. Every patient who passes through my life teaches me something. Now doctors-in-training follow me around, but I think I learn more from my students than they do from me.

Today Brooke is here. She is two years away from applying to medical school. She has a degree in natural resources from Oregon State University, but recently returned to OSU as a premedical student.

"Why did you decide to study medicine?" I ask.

"My grandma passed away in 2010. She had two doctors. One was amazing and listened to her as a person. The other treated her like a crackpot old lady and told her to take pills. I'm not saying she was an easy patient, but the difference in how she did after seeing each doctor was amazing. Her body did better on the days she saw the doctor who cared."

"What a powerful story. Have you had an opportunity to work with patients?"

"I volunteer at a hospice and the free clinic. I really enjoy it."

"You must meet a lot of wonderful doctors there."

"Not really. Doctors are on automatic pilot as they try to navigate through a staggeringly high volume of patients. It's so disheartening. And what's worse, everyone I speak with says, 'That's just the way it is. It is too expensive, difficult, and risky to go into private practice anymore. You can't be a solo doctor in this day and age.' After meeting you, I know there is another way."

"You haven't worked with solo docs?"

"No. I haven't met anyone else who has escaped our broken system to practice medicine as it should be practiced—on a personal and human level. I was worried that I was having childish delusions of grandeur by thinking I could actually practice medicine in such a way in today's climate. I worried I'd go through med school and residency only to find that in the end there was no refuge from our inhumane health care system. But hearing you speak to the premeds the other night was so inspiring. It gave me goosebumps."

"Maybe I should write a book to help premedical students. Do you mind if I include you?"

"Sure. I'm here because there are no tools or mentors to help me be the doctor I'd like to be. Several medical students have told me they haven't found any real mentors either. I feel like we are just shoved out to sea in a rowboat with no oars."

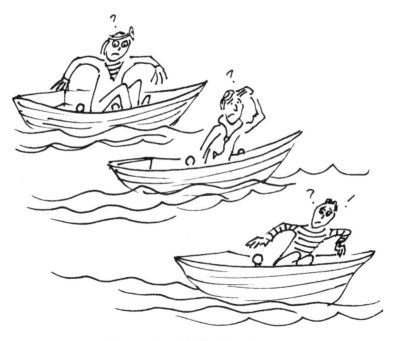

**Mentorless Medical Students**

I recall how lonely I felt as a medical student. "How sad. I thought medical education had improved since I was in school."

"Pamela, the doctors are so busy. They run around scared. It seems we should never do anything for patients outside of the clinic, as we should be terrified that patients will sue the pants off us. That's like saying don't help anyone because they might be mean sometimes. That's why I want to watch you with patients, Pamela. I want to learn how to be a real doctor who cares. You are creating a life raft for us. You survived and did not become a robot."

Now students apprentice with me the same way I apprenticed with my dad. Today I announce, "This is Brooke. She's a doctor-in-training. Do you mind if she sits here while I talk to you?" Nobody ever says no.

Brooke and I spend the afternoon together. I never imagined our small community clinic would be so exciting. Brooke doesn't follow me to the morgue, the addiction clinic, city jail, or state psychiatric hospital. My patients are not generally recovering heroin addicts, prison inmates, or suicidal schizophrenics. Our patients this afternoon are run-of-the-mill folks, compared to my dad's patients. But evidently, for Brooke, watching a doctor who cares *is* exciting.

At the end of each appointment I ask the same question my dad asked his patients: "What words of wisdom do you have for this young doctor-in-training?" Patients give lots of advice:

> Listen and never lose compassion for people; remember you are human; even doctors make mistakes; please be patient with yourself; look for health, not just disease; warm your hands; don't be afraid to use your intuition; put down the pen, turn off the computer, and then put your hands on the patient and look, listen, feel, and smell, but never judge; look your patients in the eyes; take time to mentor young people because it makes you a better person and a better professional when you take time to share what you know; and the best way to learn is to teach.

The word "doctor" is derived from the Latin word *docere*, meaning to show or teach. Doctors are really teachers. But I learned a long time ago that patients don't care what you *know* until they know that you *care*.

# 56

# What's Health Care?

"How do you define health care?" I ask this question as I travel around the nation with my handheld tape recorder. From airports to Laundromats, shopping malls, and street corners, here's how Americans define health care:

Unaffordable.
Get a prescription.
A huge scam.
Severely lacking.
The industry that has grown up around medical care.
When my concerns are fully addressed.
Providing joy and happiness.
Care of mind, body, exercise, healthy eating—things I don't do.
Someone taking care of me when I'm sick.
Getting physical, emotional, spiritual care with someone I trust.
Insurance.
It's an oxymoron in America.
Something everyone deserves, but they don't get.
A paper trail.
Corporate.
Being in touch with one's own body.
Institution of human pity.

My favorite definition comes from a man in an Oregon grocery store: heath care is a return to wholeness.

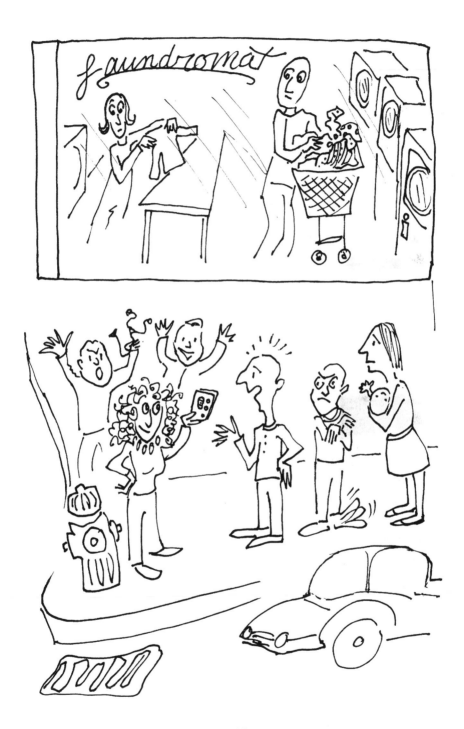

# 57

# The Vagina: A Self-Cleaning Oven

Over the years, I've been asked about the proper care and cleaning of the vagina. I wish the vagina came with an owner's manual, because lots of young women want to know how to douche and what preparations to use.

"The vagina is like a self-cleaning oven," I say.

Patients are shocked.

"Cleaning with water externally during bathing is quite adequate," I explain. "Use a small amount of mild soap if you must. Soap dries out your mucous membranes and makes them more likely to absorb toxins."

I know many young women want to smell pretty everywhere all the time, but it's not necessary and it can be harmful. For example, women reporting long-term, frequent use of talcum powder to the genital area have up to a threefold increased risk of ovarian cancer.

Women, please refrain from special preparations, perfumes, and potions. Your vagina—like your heart and liver—knows how to take care of herself as long as you don't coat her in baby powder!

Please share with anyone you know who has a vagina or loves somebody with a vagina.

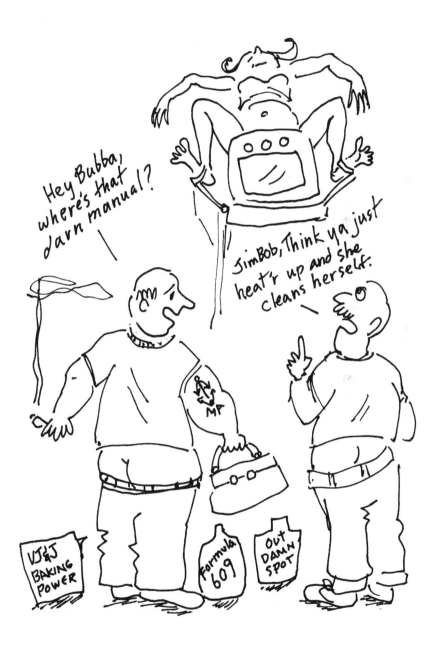

Sometimes the vagina is the smartest organ in the room.

# 58

# Self-Papping

One of my best friends, Kassy, is here for her physical. She's ten years older than I am and came of age in the '70s. She lived the free-love lifestyle. As I'm preparing to do her Pap, she says, "We used to have pelvic exam parties back in the day. We'd sit around in a big circle. Each of us was propped up on a pillow, with a mirror and our own speculum. It was like a find-your-own-cervix celebration!"

"Oh, I found myself at one of those parties a few years ago," I say. "I thought it was funny. But the other gals took it very seriously. Back in the day, did women perform their own Paps?"

Kassy laughs, "I think they did!"

As I insert the speculum into Kassy's vagina, she continues, "Hey, I know a doctor in Hawaii who did his own vasectomy in a bar."

"I used to do vasectomies, but I can't imagine doing my own in front of strangers at a bar."

"Well," Kassy replies, "you, my dear, won't be doing your own vasectomy."

"Probably right. But tell me about this guy."

"He's in med school at the time and hanging out with his friends talking vasectomies. The guys get squeamish, so he says, 'It's no big deal. I can do it on myself.' The guys say, 'Yeah, right.' So he drinks a few beers and does it."

As we finish up, I add, "I've just read about a doctor who did his own appendectomy. In the '60s on a Soviet Antarctic expedition, this Russian doctor in the middle of nowhere diagnoses himself with appendicitis. He's the only one who can do his operation, so he does. I think he uses local anesthesia, but maybe he needs a supplementary swig of vodka."

"Incredible," Kassy says.

"Kassy, you're almost due for your colonoscopy. Wanna go to the doctor who did his own colonoscopy? Just read an article about this guy. He leans forward in a chair while watching the monitor. Then he shoves a pediatric scope up his ass."

"Sounds like fun," Kassy says.

"I think he's in Japan, though."

As Kassy leaves, I realize I'm overdue for *my* Pap. I've got all the equipment. If I can't do my own Pap after what these guys did, I'm a total wuss, which by definition is a cross between a wimp and a pussy.

I'm on the exam table in the usual position. Okay, that's not gonna work. Now I'm lying on the floor laughing. If I had kept going to yoga, this position would be easier. Finally, I collect my cervical sample. Then I ride my bicycle to the lab and drop off the specimen. Definitely a lot easier than an Antarctic appendectomy!

One week later I get my results: Satisfactory sample for evaluation. Normal Pap smear. Yay!

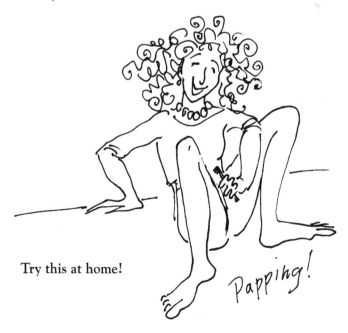

**Try this at home!**

*Papping!*

# 59

## Pap Yo Mama

Shanna is a forty-one-year-old mother who wants to stop drinking. "I've abused my body and need something to help me stop."

"Tell me more."

"Well, I just quit smoking last month. Now I want to stop drinking. My dad was an alcoholic. I drink whiskey every afternoon at four o'clock. It's a ritual. I don't want to rely on alcohol to have fun."

"Why did you start drinking?"

"I was in the middle of getting a divorce. I wasn't happy, but I loved happy hour."

"What's your plan?"

"My last drink was four days ago. I'm running again and doing yoga every day. I plan to do a juice cleanse. I'm drinking a lot of clover and nettle tea and eating organic."

"That's a great start. Shanna, when was your last Pap?"

"Six years ago, after my last child was born."

"You should come back for a Pap. Cervical cancer is preventable."

Shanna returns next week with her adorable six-year-old daughter, Kalea, in tow. Curious, Kalea follows us into the exam room to see what's going on.

"Do you mind if Kalea is in here for your exam?"

"It's fine. I delivered my three kids at home. I breastfed them until they were two. We're a close-knit family."

As I insert the speculum into Shanna's vagina, Kalea says, "Does it hurt, Mama?"

"No, baby. Mama's fine." She smiles at her daughter.

"Hey, Kalea. Look inside here. See this pink thing with the hole in the middle? It's the cervix. You used to live up inside there. And you were born out of this tiny hole!"

Kalea looks up inside her mom and smiles.

"Hey, all I'm doing is twisting this little brush. You can try."

Kalea moves the brush around and then holds it in her hand.

"Now, we swish it inside this container and we're done."

As Shanna gets dressed, I exclaim, "That was so cool! Your daughter did your Pap smear. Maybe she'll be a doctor some day."

"She's a little scientist," Shanna confirms. "She loves chasing bugs."

"Did you have fun?" Kalea smiles and shows off her live ladybug collection from her backpack.

I examine her bug collection. "Beautiful little ladies you got there, Kalea."

At the end of our sixty-minute appointment, I turn to Shanna and ask, "You haven't been drinking, have you?"

"Nope. It's been almost two weeks," she says.

"Great! Ya gotta admit this was more fun than happy hour!"

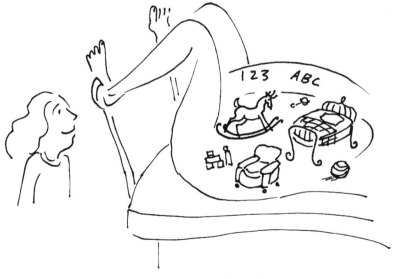

**My First Bedwomb**

# 60

## The Polyamorous Papillomavirus

Tonight I'm attending an educational symposium over dinner at an upscale restaurant. A local laboratory is sponsoring the event. The topic: human papillomavirus (HPV) testing. HPV is the most common sexually transmitted infection, and most sexually active adults have been exposed. Some strains cause genital warts. Others are linked to cancer of the cervix, vagina, vulva, penis, tonsils, tongue, and throat. It seems weird that you can kill someone you love by making love, but you can. Thankfully, the HPV vaccine should help decrease HPV-induced cancers.

There are more than 100 HPV strains and over forty of these strains may infect the human genital tract, mouth, or throat. Most people who are infected don't know they have it. People are surprised that HPV can still be transmitted even when wearing a condom.

I usually explain, "It's skin-to-skin transmission. Like shaking hands with someone who has a wart and then you get a wart. During sex, the virus can spread right where the condom ends and the skin begins—at the base of the penis as it makes contact with the genital skin of the partner."

At tonight's dinner symposium, the presenters try to simplify HPV testing guidelines. At the end of the evening, they answer questions.

I raise my hand. "How do you suggest I counsel *polyamorous* couples on their HPV risk?"

"What is a polyamorous couple?" the presenter asks.

"Polyamory means loving more than one person," I explain. "I have patients who are in intimate relationships with groups of people. All are consenting adults. I also have patients who are in *polyfidelitous* group marriages. One woman has been in a three-way marriage for ten years. I tend to counsel faithful threesomes the same as in two-person marriages. How do you suggest I counsel them?"

The presenter seems stumped. For some reason, I tend to be the one who asks the more unusual questions at medical conferences.

"So polyamorous couples can have multiple partners?" he asks.

"Yes. Married couples can be polyamorous, but it's not considered cheating because everyone is honest."

"Interesting," he says.

"As I understand it," I continue, "couples can be in a primary relationship, as in the typical two-person marriage, but they can have secondary relationships with other lovers. Sometimes they have multiple secondary relationships, also known as satellite relationships. Everything is consensual and honest."

A female physician across the room asks, "Is it like *polygamy?*"

"No. Polygamy is having more than one spouse, but polygamists' spouses are not often roaming around in satellite relationships. There are actually two forms of polygamy. Mormon polygamous sects practiced *polygyny*: multiple wives for one husband. *Polyandry* is multiple husbands for one wife, but I don't have any polyandrous patients right now."

"What about swingers?" she asks.

"For swingers, sex is like a sport. It's a recreational activity and they usually don't have emotional or spiritual attachments with one another. Sex is like shaking hands, but it feels better. Couples mix and match for the evening. While I'm no expert, I'm fascinated by what my patients tell me, and I'm just trying to figure out the best way to counsel them on HPV risk."

Dinner ends. The waitress brings me dessert. As I bite into the cherry tart, I realize there's no way for me to be obsessive-compulsive in my search for the polyamorous papillomavirus. I just need to have these folks come in for Paps and HPV testing as indicated.

While I'm all for honest, loving relationships, monogamy is a lot less work for my brain. I know it's old-fashioned, but the fall-in-love-as-two-virgins-and-get-married-for-life routine would certainly make my job easier.

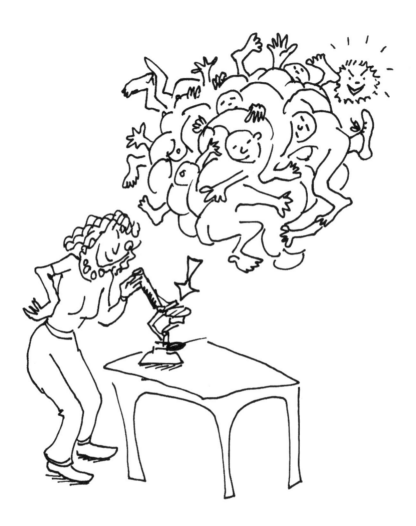

**"Aha! I found the human papillomavirus.
It's under that guy's foot!"**

Human papillomavirus can cause plantar warts on the soles of the feet. But don't worry! The HPV strains that infect the feet are not the same strains that cause genital warts or sexually transmitted cancers of the vulva, vagina, penis, anus, and throat.

# 61

# Fear Full

Beth is a twenty-five-year-old mother of twins. She suffers from anxiety and panic attacks.

Today she reports, "On the anxiety meds, I have less heart racing. I'm starting to be able to calm myself down. The meditation exercise you taught me has really helped. I'm no longer thinking negative thoughts about my family and myself. I still get nightmares. I sleep about three hours, but then wake up with an adrenaline rush and shakes. Part of the problem is I'm still nursing. I just can't stop worrying about my girls, Pamela."

"What exactly do you worry about?"

"Everything. I turn on the news and worry about tornados even though we don't have tornados here. I worry about the girls dying in a car accident, a house fire."

I spend a lot of time teaching patients to overcome their fears. Today I explain, "Beth, we live in a fear-driven culture. There's always gonna be something to worry about. For example, I just went to Staples for office supplies." I reach into my desk and retrieve an unopened package of letter openers. "I got these square-plastic letter openers. The back of the package reads: 'CAUTION: Blades are extremely sharp. Safety goggles recommended.'"

Beth laughs, "For a letter opener? But that's ridiculous! Don't worry, Pamela. The razor is embedded inside."

"I know. But just to be safe, I have protection." I reach into my drawer and put on my safety goggles. "Now I'm ready to open my mail."

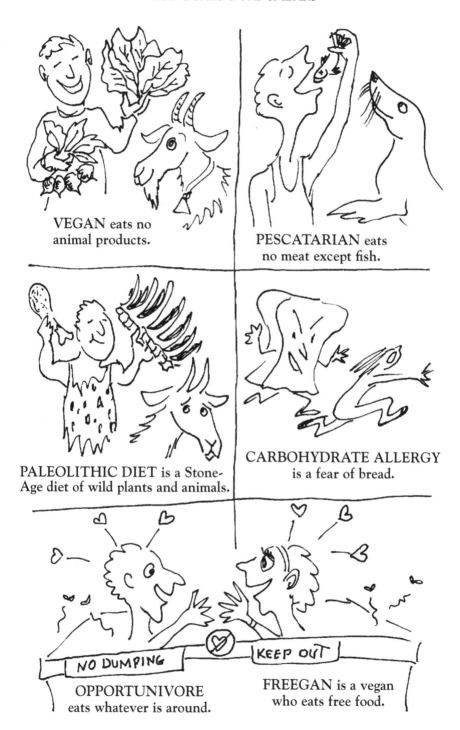

VEGAN eats no animal products.

PESCATARIAN eats no meat except fish.

PALEOLITHIC DIET is a Stone-Age diet of wild plants and animals.

CARBOHYDRATE ALLERGY is a fear of bread.

NO DUMPING

KEEP OUT

OPPORTUNIVORE eats whatever is around.

FREEGAN is a vegan who eats free food.

# 62

# The Best Diet

I've been mostly vegan since medical school. Back then almost nobody had a special diet. That was in Texas. Now I'm in Oregon, where all my patients have peculiar dietary requirements.

I take care of the woman who claims she's allergic to carbohydrates. And the proud pescatarian man. Oh, and the opportunivore who fell in love with the freegan.

I've got a vegan raw-foodist family. The parents just divorced with split custody. Dad adopted the paleo diet. Now the kids enjoy kale smoothies and cashew-carob-coconut balls by week and eat like cavemen on the weekends.

My newest patient is a heavy woman who won't eat any fruits or vegetables—except mushrooms.

"So what do you eat?" I ask.

"A large bowl of ice cream at least once or twice a day and sometimes for breakfast. And I'm not gonna quit."

"Okay."

"Any idea how I can lose thirty pounds?" she asks.

"Umm . . . I'm thinking expand your mushroom intake. Have you gotten into portobellos or chanterelles?"

I try to make things simple for patients, but I find people are more confused than ever about what to eat. At the grocery store, I understand why. Everything is gluten-free and twice as expensive. There are gluten-free chips and salsa, gluten-free ice cream, gluten-free cupcakes and cookies.

Maybe the best diet is *glutton*-free.

# 63

# Medical Disintermediation

Anita, a retired medical social worker, believes an ideal clinic would "eliminate the medical assistant who weighs and measures and takes notes that the physician doesn't read anyway." Reviewing Anita's town hall testimony, I realize her request can be summarized in one word: disintermediation—removing the middleman.

Doctors didn't always have staff. Back in the 1950s, there was no billing department, no referral clerk, no lead receptionist, and no medical assistant. Most doctors did everything on their own.

My dad started out as a general practitioner in a little neighborhood clinic. He kept all his medical records on index cards in a recipe box on his

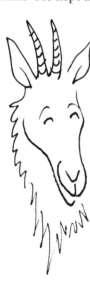

desk. And he looked at patients, not a computer screen. Back then doctors did house calls. Maybe that was ideal health care.

Fast forward sixty years and I realize I'm practicing medicine kind of like my dad—minus the index cards.

I'm a solo-solo doc—that's solo with no staff.

Some physicians may need employees. I don't. On occasion I ask my patients, "If I had a secretary waiting for you, a medical assistant sitting between us, a coder huddled in the corner, and a few other doctors rushing down the hall, would you feel you were getting better care?"

They laugh and beg me not to change.

# 64

# Idiopathic

Patients want to know what's going on. The problem is, much of the time, doctors don't know. Fortunately, we have a diagnosis for that. "Idiopathic" is a medical term that means arising spontaneously from an unknown cause. In other words, idiopathic means we don't understand why you have what you have.

For example, a patient arrives with a seizure disorder of unknown cause. Diagnosis: idiopathic epilepsy. Another patient has a crooked spine and we have no idea why. Diagnosis: idiopathic scoliosis. Patients feel relieved to know the diagnosis even if the diagnosis means we don't know. But patients don't know we don't know.

Today I'm on the phone with a cardiologist discussing a mutual patient with idiopathic cardiomyopathy, when he asks, "Do you know what that means?"

I respond, "Idiopathic cardiomyopathy means the heart muscles are not functioning properly and we don't know why."

He says, "No, I mean the word 'idiopathic.'"

I pause.

"Idiopathic," he retorts, "means the doctor is an idiot and the patient is pathetic."

# 65

# The Claim Game

I find most insurance companies easy to deal with. Not this one.

With most insurers, I treat the patient, submit the claim, and they send a check. But not this insurance company. Since merging with a larger health plan, they stopped paying all my claims. But they're still collecting monthly premiums from my patients.

When doctors sign contracts with insurance companies, we agree to their rules and reimbursement rates. We're not allowed to bill patients. So if the insurer doesn't pay, we work for free. And since it's not so easy to get out of these contracts, we're screwed.

Today, I'm back on the phone with the bad insurance company. I've called so often the women know me by name. On hold, I hear, "This call will be recorded for quality assurance."

A woman picks up. "Hi, this is Kacey. How may I help you?"

"It's me again. Dr. Wible. Still no payments, Kacey. I appreciate you trying to help me get paid. Your new employer is behaving unethically. You probably have people screaming at you all day long. I guess you're probably looking for other employment."

"Yeah, some of the gals are leaving."

"Do you really think I should pursue these unpaid claims? I don't have time to sit on the phone all day calling a bunch of 1-800 numbers."

Kacey checks in with her cohorts. They agree that it would be a hassle.

"Okay. Thanks. I won't waste my time."

In her bubbly voice, Kacey asks, "Is there anything else I can do for you today?"

I laugh. "The only thing I want is to get out of this contract before my fortieth birthday."

Three days later, a large turquoise envelope arrives by certified mail at my office. I open it. "From All of Us! HAPPY BIRTHDAY!" Wow. It's a birthday card from all my new friends at the call center, with a canceled contract enclosed.

The next month, payments for my previously submitted claims start flowing in.

I guess it pays to be nice.

# 66

# Tribute to a Cowboy Doctor

After two decades of formal education, today I'm finally set loose with real patients. It's the actual moment I've been waiting for my entire life.

We're each assigned to a family doc for the month. I scroll down the list of third-year medical students, place my right index finger beside my name, slide it across the page, then read aloud: *E. Sinks McLarty, Jr., M.D., III.*

The next morning I find his office—a small nondescript building with his name on the side—and enter the waiting room, which features 1970s-style wood paneling, faded and covered with the grime of decades of cigarette smoke. Centrally located is a large oil portrait of E. Sinks McLarty, Sr., M.D., who opened the place nearly 100 years ago. I pass rows of empty chairs to the front desk, where I meet three bouncy women—all relatives of Dr. McLarty. I introduce myself to the friendly, frenzied group of chatty chart finders, then the garrulous gang scurries me down a narrow, smoke-filled hallway where I meet Dr. McLarty's nurse, affectionately nicknamed "Olive Oyl."

A friendly, slender, snappy-tongued woman with a gravelly voice, Olive Oyl chain-smokes at her desk. Her deep red lipstick and nail polish are the color of freshly clotted blood. She escorts me into a dimly lit room where I'm not at all sure I'm safe. There, on the couch, I meet Dr. McLarty—a seventy-year-old cowboy eating Metamucil wafers while puffing on a pipe. He wears Wrangler corduroys and sports a crew cut with some gray hairs shooting through. With his thick Texas twang, he slurs his words together around southern *slangisms* and medical anecdotes.

With pen, paper, and stethoscope, I follow Dr. McLarty around to see what I can glean from him. I'm immediately struck by his speech with patients. He calls all the men "*pahdna*" and all the women "*shuga*." Isn't that sexual harassment?

Dr. McLarty has no tolerance for big-government rules. When a patient needs a triplicate form signed, he snaps, "Well, now, shuga, that's a bunch of horseshit!" or "I don't give a ram dam or a rat's butt!" While cursing, he signs the forms, gives one to the patient, and throws the other two across the room in a wad. "Hell, I'll make toilet paper out of it one day," he rambles as he tramps out of the room.

Dr. McLarty makes even the common cold an event to remember. "Okay, now, pahdna, let's look in that there snoot. Ah, a little redness, nothing to say grace over. Let's listen to your ticker while I gotcha here." Slamming down the chart, he exclaims, "You've prob'ly got some of that damn crud we've seen going around!"

In the next room, an elderly woman complains of joint pain. His diagnosis: "You've got arthritis! Well, hell, you can see that. No need to pay for that, shuga. Now hold that cane in your left hand and tell Byron to give ya a damn golf ball to carry around in the right." He didn't cure her arthritis, but she looked like an avid golfer when she left.

After seeing a few patients in the morning, Dr. McLarty closes down for a two-hour lunch. We all squeeze into his office on the couch to watch soap operas. During a romantic interracial scene, they shake their heads in unison. "Oh, no! We don't believe in that!"

So I offer the clan some of my chocolate soy ice cream and one gal gasps, "Oh, no! My husband wouldn't like that!" Dr. McLarty puts down his Metamucil wafer and grabs a spoonful. "That's pretty darn good!"

After lunch we're getting ready to see a man named "Sunshine." Before entering the exam room, Dr. McLarty pulls me aside and says, "This family's been shot in the damn butt with bad luck!"

"What's going on?" I ask.

"He got cancer. I've known a week, but gonna break it to him now."

"Why didn't you tell him last week?" I ask.

"If he lived by himself, I'd a told 'im right away this is how the cow ate the cabbage, but his wife, Lordy, ya couldn't scrape her off the wall last night," he rants as he trudges down the hall.

I gathered that Sunshine's wife was extremely anxious.

We enter the room. Doc pats the old fellow on the shoulder and says, "Sunshine, now I ain't gonna pull any punches by tellin' ya we got a drug." After a few cryptic sentences, he asks, "Ya get what I'm sayin'?"

Sunshine replies, "Yep! Lights out."

That was the entire office visit.

Most of Doc McLarty's patients are old white guys who have aged right alongside him. But this afternoon, we jump into Doc's old pickup to see a young gal in the hospital. On exam, he notices her breast implants and asks, "Hey now, shuga, how long ya had these damn things blown up that way?" She answers politely and the interview continues without a hitch.

We only saw one kid that month. As the boy raced around the exam room, Dr. McLarty quickly warned, "Hey now, pahdna, get back up there on that there table. We don't want ya to bust your gazoo!"

I'll always savor my month with E. Sinks McLarty, Jr., M.D., III. I didn't learn much about diagnosing or treating disease, but I learned a lot about human relationships and the art of medical practice.

I sure miss him.

So, after fifteen years, I track him down to thank him.

He answers on the first ring.

With my heart pounding, I ask, "Is this really Dr. McLarty?"

"Yep, this is Doctor McLarty. Who the hell is this?" he shouts.

"I'm a medical student you mentored long ago, and I just want to say thank you."

"Well, thank you, sweetie, but I got cancer of the bladder and just had therapy today, and I'm bleedin' like hell!" Before I can express my sympathy, he quickly blurts out, "What comes around goes around. Thanks for calling on me, but I gotta go pee again!"

He hangs up on me.

That's it.

I never even tell him my name—not sure he would have remembered me—but I do get to thank him before lights out.

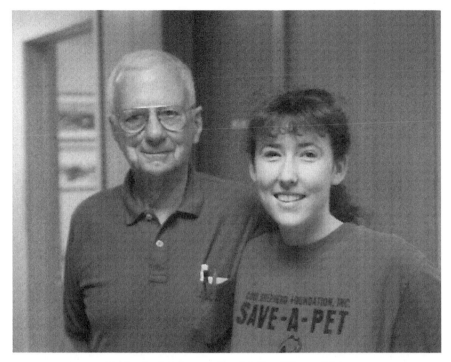

**E. Sinks McLarty, Jr., M.D., III, and Me**

# 67

# The Good Old Days

My dad is eighty-eight years old. He finally retired from medicine at eighty-six. I call to check on him. "What are you up to, Dad?"

"I just returned from synagogue a few hours ago. Right now I'm catching up on my reading. I'm finishing up the fiftieth anniversary issue of *Medical Economics*.

That's Dad living it up on a Saturday night.

"It came out in 1973," he continues. "It's a nostalgic look at the U.S. physician from 1923—the year I was born—through 1973. I'll mail it to you when I'm done."

One week later, I read all 302 pages on Saturday evening. In a partial reprint of the first article from October 1923, Dr. Royal S. Copeland—then junior U.S. Senator from New York—suggests America would be better off if more doctors entered politics. He writes:

> Most of the government's vital problems have to do with things more familiar to the physician than to anybody else in society. . . . The doctor is better qualified to know the desires and necessities of the human family than the lawyer, the engineer, and even the priest. . . . He is an eyewitness to the suffering of the poor. . . . In consequence his soul is moved and he becomes an advocate of social justice.

I agree with Copeland's sentiment. It *is* the physician who is in the best position to heal the wounds of a nation. But the mission of *Medical*

*Economics* is not to turn every physician into a social activist. Its mission is to educate physicians on the business of medicine.

Nearly ninety years after the journal's debut, physicians have the same concerns they had in the 1920s. Doctors still fear an imminent doctor shortage. They still suffer from a lack of business education. They still believe high-paying specialties will force the solo family doc into extinction.

In the 1920s came the group practice, and the 1930s brought a trend toward salaried jobs. In the 1940s, government, labor, and business groups continued to erode solo doctors' "rugged individualism." Over the decades, physicians have been pressured to see more and more patients. Even house calls were nixed as financially unwise.

Many doctors miss the good old days. In 1973, one old doc lamented, "Medical offices are just mills." Oh no! I wonder what he'd say today!

Physicians across the country are now contacting *me* for business advice: "Is it really possible to go solo? How can you do house calls? And your own billing? Is it hard? Can you serve the poor and not go out of business? How do you work without staff? And be available 24/7?"

Yes, I accept insurance and I never turn anyone away for lack of money. I love doing house calls. With low overhead, I can work less and earn more than I ever made as an employed physician. Technology makes it easy to do my own billing. Maintaining clear boundaries with patients, I don't need staff to protect me from patients.

One evening, I ask my mom for her advice on why doctors keep asking me for advice.

Mom is seventy-one years old. She's a retired psychiatrist. She had a thriving private practice in the 1970s and '80s in Dallas.

"Mom, how did you do it?"

"My entire philosophy is self-sufficiency. I gather information and figure things out on my own."

I recite a list of questions doctors keep asking me.

She says, "What's wrong with them? It's common sense. They need to go off by themselves, spend a few hours thinking about these problems, and come up with a solution."

"What's your best business advice?"

"Have a patient base. Don't be fearful. Figure out how to do your own billing. Immediately incorporate to save on taxes. Get a good CPA—preferably Jewish. I've had the best luck with Jewish CPAs. They perform miracles."

"In solo practice," she continues, "I earned twice as much as the guys. Most doctors are risk-averse and afraid. They want to be taken care of by a hospital system."

"Mom, how come smart people can be taken advantage of so easily? Docs still believe they can't succeed in solo practice. Why?"

"Well, in psychiatry, most doctors had psychiatric reasons for not succeeding. They were fearful. They didn't believe in themselves. Seemed like they had no confidence in their ability to succeed. I found psychiatrists to be anxious, scared, and lacking self-confidence."

"How did medicine change in the 1980s?"

"In the '80s, corporations brainwashed us. They overtook us. I blame doctors. Doctors don't think for themselves. They just follow along. I saw what corporations were doing and I didn't want to play their game, so I went into solo practice. And my CPA and I did really well."

"Any other advice for doctors today?"

"Have confidence. Ask yourself: Do I believe in myself? Okay. Then find an office and hire a CPA."

The solo family doc isn't extinct. I'm proof of that. I believe the good old days are here now. And the best days in medicine are yet to come.

I'm with Senator Copeland. I believe it *is* the physician who is best qualified to heal the individual patient and the entire community. It is still the physician who is eyewitness to the suffering of the poor. And it is still the physician whose soul is moved to be an advocate for social justice. Now is the perfect time for doctors to start community clinics, to work as social activists, and to become political leaders. America is waiting.

I think doctors need to believe in themselves a little more and maybe follow my mom's advice—find a good CPA.

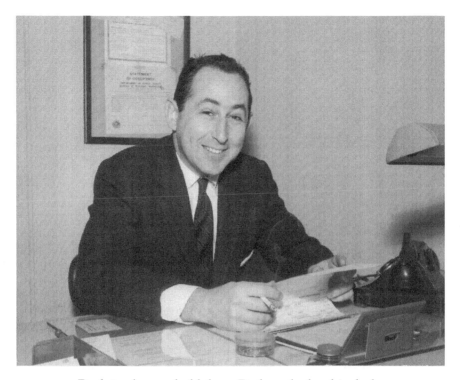

Back in the good old days, Dad smoked at his desk.
(So did all the doctors!)

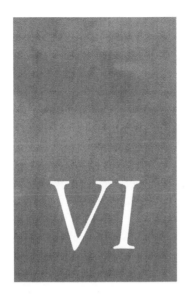

# On Intuition

*Sometimes answers arise spontaneously*
*from mysterious places*
*and then—without warning—*
*the perfect words fly right out of my mouth.*
*It seems weird,*
*but I've diagnosed and cured many patients*
*without really thinking.*

# 68

# Speak Your Truth

Sequoia is a sixteen-year-old who is having difficulty holding her urine.

"When did it start?" I ask.

"About a month ago when we moved to my dad's girlfriend's house."

"How's it going there?"

"Well, I live in this room detached from her house. When I go in the main house, they're usually arguing. It's not great."

"How's the rest of your life?"

"Umm . . . kind of a mixed bag. I don't like most people at school. Kids at school annoy me. I only have two really good friends."

"So tell me about your urine problems."

"I go to the bathroom to pee, like, three or four times a night. I never had this happen before. It's weird."

"Does your urine smell funny? Does it burn when you pee?"

"Not really."

"Any blood?"

"Nope."

"How much water are you drinking?" I ask.

"Like normal."

"Does it happen during the day?"

"I don't really have this peeing problem at my friend's house or at school."

I don't examine her. I don't even ask for a urine specimen. I write Sequoia one prescription: "Speak your truth."

And I explain, "If the adults in your home are making you feel uncomfortable, you need to tell them. Always express yourself. Don't clam up. Your bladder is trying to tell you something."

One week later I call Sequoia to see how she is doing. She says, "I told my dad I'm pissed with him. Now my urine problems are gone. Thanks."

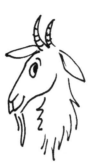

# 69

# Paper Cut

It's fall 2002. I've spent nearly two years working at a small clinic in Olympia, Washington—home of the uninspired and overinsured state worker. Many of my patients are employed by the state and they seem bored out of their minds. They love to tell me how much they hate their jobs and often take time off in the middle of their workweek just to do so.

Sue comes back in today.

"So what brings you in, Sue?"

"I need to open a workers' compensation case for a work-related injury," she claims.

"What's going on?" I ask.

She unravels several layers of bandages from her left middle finger and then grimaces as she peels off a Band-Aid from the tip. "I've got a paper cut," she says.

I look closely at her finger. "I don't see anything, Sue." She points back to the tip of her finger. I look closer.

Intuitively, I blurt out, "Sue, do you have any idea how many people will get paper cuts from dealing with your paperwork for a workers' comp claim on a paper cut?" I usher her back to work.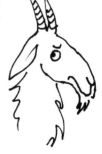

Incredible. I could never make this stuff up.

# 70

# Medical Aquarium Warning

Many busy clinics display a large fish tank in the waiting room. Staring at fish can help patients relax and lower blood pressure and anxiety before appointments. But how do fish feel about staring at miserable patients all day long?

In the fall of 1999, an exotic eel makes his feelings known. One morning he jumps out of the tank, flinging himself across the waiting room.

A kind older man picks up the eel; that's when the eel attacks him.

When I arrive at work, the poor man is in the procedure room, with doctors pulling the eel off his finger while the clinic manager is on the phone with the malpractice carrier. I'm not sure whether we have liability coverage for eel attacks.

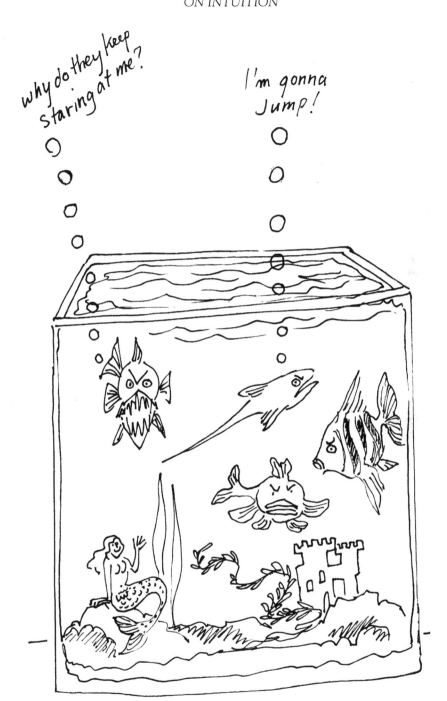

**Mad Fish Disease**

# 71

# Adventure in Hypochondria

Helen is an overinsured hypochondriac. During the last two years, she has tried to convince me to diagnose her with five fatal diseases. I spend most of my time talking her out of expensive tests and reassuring her that she's fine.

Today, Helen is back. As soon as I enter the exam room, she says, "I fell in the tub this morning. I've fractured my back."

"Let me take a look." I examine her and find a small area of tenderness along the mid-thoracic spine over her vertebrae. "It's probably not a fracture."

Helen demands an X-ray, "just to be sure." This time I give in.

The radiologist calls right back.

"How does it look?" I ask. "No fracture, right?"

"No fracture, but she has cancer. Her lungs are full of metastases."

"What!?" I exclaim. "Don't say anything to Helen. Just send her back immediately with the films. I'll talk to her."

While Helen's waiting in the exam room, I review her X-rays on the light box in my office. Very interesting pattern of disease, evenly spaced lesions in groups of three. They look like tiny flower petals.

I return to the exam room where Helen eagerly awaits the bad news. She's sitting on the exam table in the most beautiful purple shirt covered with evenly spaced, tiny metallic flower petals.

Helen says, "It's bad news, Doc. I fractured my spine."

"I see you kept your shirt on for the X-ray."

"Yes, Doctor. I did."

"Helen. You're as healthy as a horse."

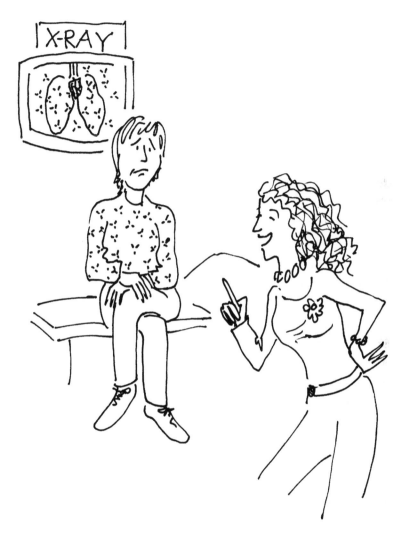

Sometimes the only diagnosis is "flower petals."

# 72

## Lonnie's Earwax

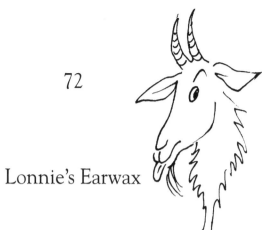

Lonnie has seen me for five years. He's a good guy. Always pays his bills. He works as a videographer and tours with big rock-and-roll bands like KISS and Aerosmith. Now he's out of work and struggling.

Two years ago, Lonnie referred his friend, Cheryl, to me. She lives in Los Angeles, but now she comes up to Oregon for medical care. Today, Cheryl calls: "Lonnie has an appointment with you tomorrow, and I know he is without funds. I'll pay for his visit. I'd pay in person, but I'm in L.A. I'll pop the check in the mail today. I hope this will work for you."

"I'm impressed, Cheryl. Why are you doing this?"

"Lonnie and I have been good friends through thick and thin. I've always been there for him and he for me—that's why. He has had a really rough couple of years. I'm trying to help him find work."

The next day, Lonnie enters the office.

"Hey Lonnie, Cheryl is covering your visit."

"What did you say, Doc? Think my ears are plugged up again."

I irrigate his ears and remove a lot of impacted wax.

"Any idea why I keep getting so much wax?" he asks.

"Nope. No idea."

On his way out Lonnie says, "Guess what, Doc? In two months, I got a gig with Def Leppard!"

"Wear ear plugs or you'll go deaf, Lonnie! Wait! I've got a feeling you do need all that wax. Let me grab that big chunk out of the trash. I'll put it in this container and you can take it to the concert."

# 73

# Aerotoxic Syndrome

Dan, a sixty-three-year-old diabetic, is here with his wife, Barbara.

"We just got back from visiting our new granddaughter in Washington, D.C., but Dan got sick on the flight," Barbara says.

Dan adds, "We sat on the runway a long time. It was hot and the fumes were intense. In flight I recall hearing 'We're at 10,000 feet,' and suddenly I got sweats and nausea. I was clammy, light-headed. So I checked my blood sugar, but it was normal."

"And then he passed out," says Barbara. "He slumped over and then arched his back, like he was having a seizure. His eyes rolled back in his head. He made gurgling sounds and fell forward. He was in and out of consciousness for the entire three-hour flight. Every once in a while Dan lifted his head to say, 'Well, I'm still here.' It was scary."

"At least I kept my sense of humor," Dan chuckles.

"Then what happened?"

"He came to at 20,000 feet as we descended into Portland. We rolled him to the baggage claim in a wheelchair."

"I felt normal when I left the airport," Dan shares. "And I've been fine since."

"Did you seek medical attention on the plane?" I ask Dan.

"I wanted to ask for a doctor, but I couldn't get the words out."

"We needed a doctor or some oxygen," Barbara adds, "but all they gave us was some orange juice and a coke."

"My first diagnosis: you're too nice, Barbara. You've been living in Oregon too long. You gotta act like you're from New Jersey."

"But I *am* from New Jersey."

"Well, you gotta act like it. Be aggressive. Grab a flight attendant. Scream for help."

I check Dan out. "Everything is perfect on your exam and EKG. You do have a high resting heart rate that may have predisposed you to the event. Possible diagnoses include aerotoxic syndrome caused by jet fuel toxins that can contaminate air circulating in planes. Altitude sickness may be a problem too, as cabin pressures are often maintained at the equivalent of 8,000 feet or so."

Dan turns to Barbara.

Intuitively, I explain, "It's like you were climbing Mount Everest while breathing jet fumes."

"We're going on a trip in a few months," Dan says. "How should we prepare?"

"Well, if all they're going to do is give you orange juice, you better bring your own oxygen monitor, a blood pressure machine, and a mask to protect you from vapors. And Barb, you need to practice being a little more bitchy and demanding."

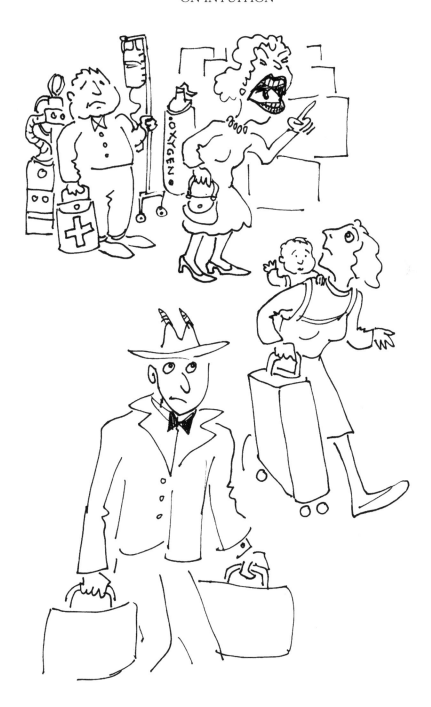

**Diabetic Dan and Bitchy Barb board their next flight.**

# 74

# The Big Dripper

Chris brings his wife to the office. "You got to help her, Doc."

"What's happening?"

"She can't sleep. She's up all night, tearing her clothes off, opening all the windows. She can't sit still. I love Rachel, Doc. Been married since '89, but she's driving me bonkers."

"So, Rachel, when did all this start?"

Before Rachel can answer, Chris says, "It's happening now. Starts right here at the base of her neck." Chris strokes Rachel's neck and shows me his wet fingers. Beads of sweat are dripping down her forehead. In minutes her shirt is soaked.

I grab the Kleenex and blot her dry with marginal success.

"It happens every ten minutes," Rachel says, "all day long. I just lost my job 'cause I'm always running for towels. I can't think straight and it sets off my panic attacks."

"Maybe it's time for estrogen."

They agree.

Rachel calls a few days later. "Doing better, Doc. I'm down to once an hour now, but around three o'clock in the afternoon I get the big dripper."

The following week, a police officer directs Rachel back to my office. Frazzled, she explains, "An hour ago, driving through a construction zone, I got the big one. I sped up to make it through there real quick, before the panic set in. The police chased me down. By the time the cop got to my car, I was drenched."

"Then what?"

"He told me to get right in to see my doctor. He wanted me to tell you that he thinks my hot flashes are very serious."

"Hmm . . . how about we double your estrogen and see what trouble you can get into next week."

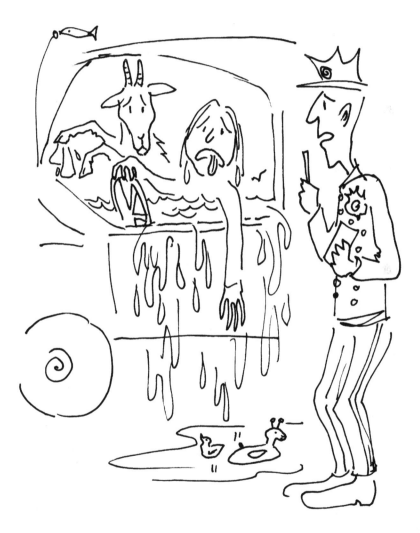

**DUIE = Driving Under Inadequate Estrogen**

# 75

# Allergic to Sex

Kate is a happily married woman in her forties. She has an awesome husband. Great kids. They're in college now. Kate's tubes are tied. She's done having kids. Today she's here for her physical.

"So how's everything going?"

"Wonderful. I got a promotion at work. And my oldest daughter graduates this year."

"Anything you're concerned about?"

"Lately, after sex, I have intense burning and itching in my vagina and it can last hours. Sometimes a long bath helps."

I have a feeling she has developed an allergy to her husband. "Do you ever have wheezing or hives?"

"No."

We continue talking as I complete her exam. "Kate, everything looks perfect in your vagina. I know this may sound strange, but I think you're allergic to your husband's semen. Some women have more serious reactions, but I've not heard of any fatalities."

"But we've been married twenty years. Why now?"

"It can happen at any time. Nobody knows why. It's more common in people who have other allergies."

"What shall we do?" she asks.

"Abstinence? Just kidding. Try an antihistamine before intercourse. If that doesn't help, I think you're back to condoms. Here's an epinephrine kit just in case you get a life-threatening reaction. And no oral sex!"

"My husband's gonna love this one."

Kate comes back a month later. "Condoms are working best, but is there anything else we can do?"

"You can see an allergist. Diagnosis is with a skin-prick test using your husband's semen. Treatment options include desensitizing injections containing fresh, diluted semen. Or, you can have increasing concentrations of his semen inserted in your vagina—under physician supervision, of course."

"So my husband masturbates into a cup and the nurse runs down the hall with it and then the doctor pours it into my vagina?"

"Yes! And you'll need to have sex at least three times every week for the treatments to work. If you skip a week, your vagina might start burning again."

"Well, my husband will love that part of the treatment."

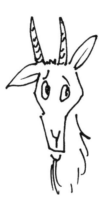

# 76

# The War on Pubic Hair

Over the years, I've noticed a lot of stubbly pits and pubes during Paps. Women apologize for the stubble, for not having freshly shaven legs. They usually start their exams with an apology, such as: "I didn't get a chance to shave my armpits. They're so sweaty. Sorry you have to touch 'em"; or "Oh no! Sorry about the stubble. I forgot to shave my legs."

My response is always the same: "What? Why apologize for hair?"

Hair insulates and offers a buffer to chafing and abrasions. Shaving inflames follicles, leaving microscopic cuts that act as a breeding ground for nasty bacteria like staph, herpes, or other sexually transmitted infections. There's also the risk of abscesses, boils, and deeper infections that necessitate surgery on one's genitals or inner thighs. Some claim shaving their pubes increases sexual sensitivity. My plea: just a trim, not a clear-cut.

I live in Oregon now. My patients are mostly happy and hairy. I prefer the natural look. I love all the smiley women with hairy pits who never apologize for not shaving their legs.

Interestingly, men arrive for their exams sometimes sweaty, really hairy, and often overweight. Not once in my career do I recall a man ever apologizing for his hair, his smell, or anything about his body during his exam.

Maybe the war goes beyond pubic hair. Maybe women are at war with themselves.

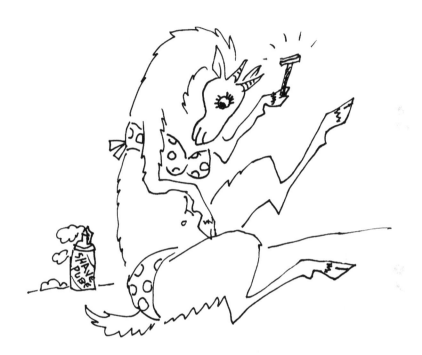

# 77

# Penis Problems

Over the years, I've heard women say, "I'd never go to a male gynecologist. How would he know how my body works?" If that's the case, maybe I'm not the right person to handle penis problems. But every day, men come in with their penises, and they want to discuss their problems. Having never owned or operated one, I try my best.

Bob—a friend and patient—is in for erectile dysfunction. He's involved in a new relationship with a woman whom I know. We talk about some of the fun new pills that may work for him. Since he's uninsured, I guide him toward the least expensive option.

This afternoon, Bob calls to alert me, "I got a partial fill on my prescription today. I fully expected it to be expensive because we all know that the pharmaceutical industry is a big rip-off. But I was nonetheless shocked to pay twenty-four dollars for one pill. Shall I give you a report on how my expensive new drug works tonight?"

"Yes, please."

His morning e-mail reads:

> Honestly, we had better sex the morning after the drug had presumably worn off. We're still quite new at this and are figuring out what works for us. As a sensitive New-Age guy, I like to try to stretch it out to show her the best possible time, but from the standpoint of enjoying intercourse, what seems to work best is to keep foreplay to a minimum

and just get in there before the erection starts to fizzle out. This aging shit is getting old.

Maybe the magic pill was anticlimactic. I could try a few more drugs on Bob, but I have a feeling he might get better advice from a man with real-world experience—maybe a male gynecologist.

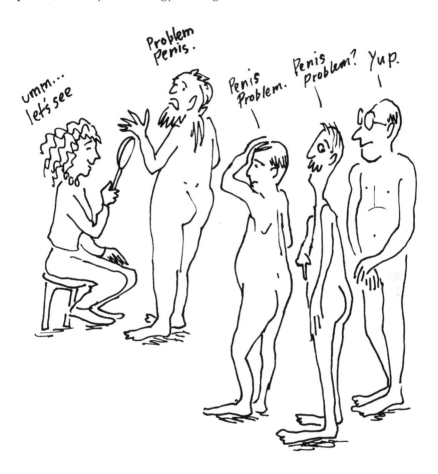

Penis Problems

# 78

# Joe—Part One

Joe has smoked two packs per day since his teens. He knows better. I don't need to lecture him on the dangers of smoking.

"I was a respiratory therapist back in Brooklyn," Joe says in his thick New York accent.

"And you smoked?"

"Yep. All the respiratory therapists smoked, Doc."

"Reminds me of cardiologists who order bacon and eggs in the hospital cafeteria, but then tell patients to eat low-cholesterol diets."

Joe continues, "It's my anxiety. That's why I smoke. I moved to Oregon a few years ago for the quiet life. I'm gonna turn my life around. You'll see, Doc."

Today we're celebrating. Joe hasn't had a cigarette since he went into the hospital last month with pneumonia.

"I feel terrific!" he says. "I've turned the corner, Doc."

The next day I'm bicycling through town. I turn at the corner of Sixth Avenue. To my right, I see a man smoking a cigarette. I have a feeling it's Joe. He's standing next to an apartment complex. I get closer. Oblivious, he has headphones on and he's tapping his left hand on his thigh. So I speed up and then stop suddenly right in front of his face. The high-pitched squeal from my brake pads startles him.

He does a tough guy pose and tries to stare me down. "What's your problem?" he says.

I lean my bicycle against the door to his apartment.

"Who are you?" he demands as he closes in on me.

We're in a standoff. He takes off his headphones. I take off my bike helmet. He removes the cigarette from his mouth. I remove the sunglasses from my face.

Then he slinks back against the building and almost cries, "Oh my God. Oh no. Oh no. Oh my God. I can't believe it. I promise this is the first cigarette. I just picked it up just now. It's the first one. I mean the last one. I promise I'm going to quit, Doc. I'll quit now, tonight, as soon as you leave. It's the last one. I promise. I can't believe it's you. What is this? Why are you here? What are you, an angel?"

I put my hand on top of Joe's balding head, look straight into his eyes, and I bless him: "Your life has been spared one more day."

Then I ride off into the sunset.

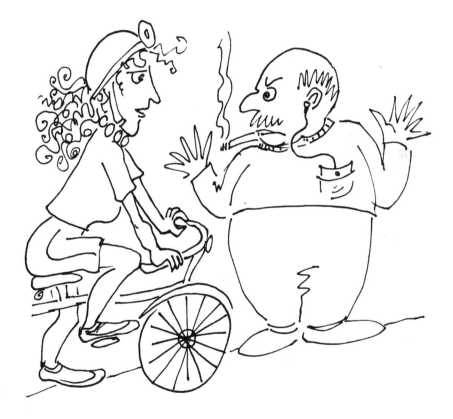

# 79

# Joe—Part Two

Joe just had open-heart surgery. A triple bypass. When he left the hospital last month, he promised he'd follow a healthy diet and quit smoking for good. I call to review his cholesterol results. He picks up on the second ring.

"Hold on a minute," he says.

The reception is poor, but I can make out a few people talking. I hear the muffled voice of a woman.

"Okay, so you want a combo meal, sir? That's a BK Bacon Triple Cheeseburger, large fries, and a large Coke. Anything else, sir?"

"Can you change that to a Diet Coke?"

"Okay. That will be $7.29 at the window."

"Sorry, who is this again?" he asks.

"It's Dr. Wible."

"Oh my God. Oh no. Oh no. Oh my God. I can't believe it. I promise this is the first burger since the bypass. It's just a treat. It's the first time, I promise. I've been eating more salads. I was even vegetarian for a few days. I can't believe it's you. I can't believe you're calling now. Oh my God."

"Joe, your cholesterol is still high. You better stay on your statin. In fact, let's double the dose. You know, the drive-thru is just a shortcut to the Pearly Gates."

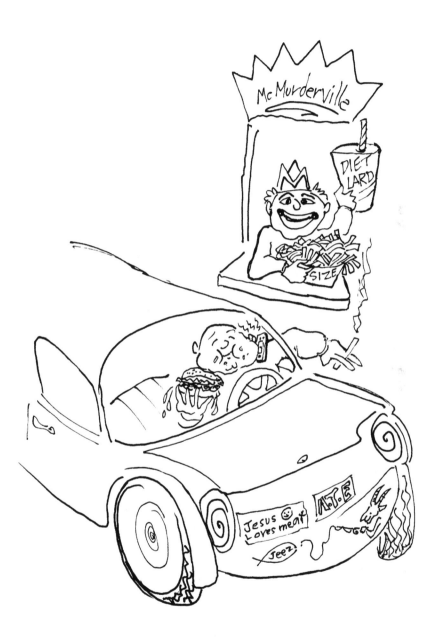

**Joe's bypass bypasses his problems.**

# 80

# Joe—Part Three

Joe comes in for refills. I usually spend thirty minutes with him. We review his cholesterol, pulmonary, and anxiety medications. Then I check in with him on his diet, smoking, and alcohol intake. Somewhere in there, he usually tells me he hates his job. Lately he complains about how difficult it is to walk from the parking lot to work without stopping to catch his breath.

As I start to speak, Joe says, "Don't waste your breath, Doc. Just give me the drugs."

I refill his prescriptions in silence.

He leaves.

I spend the evening ruminating on Joe. Was his request kind-hearted or disrespectful? I could hear the shame in his voice. His appointment was easy. No resistance. I just did what he said. Disturbed, I call Joe the next morning.

"Do you know what you're asking me to do?

"What, Doc?"

"When you asked me not to waste my breath?"

"Doc, you know I like you a lot. I just wanted to give you a break."

"Oh, I thought you were asking me to stop caring about you, Joe. You know you can't ask me to stop caring about you. That's part of my job, Joe. I'm going to care about you even if you stop caring about yourself."

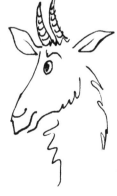

# 81

## Joe—The Final Chapter

I've taken care of Joe for seven years. He still smokes, drinks, and eats crappy food. I summarize our lack of progress and ask, "So what's going on, Joe?"

"I'm ready to move on, Doc. But I'm not courageous enough to commit suicide. Ya see, I'm Catholic. If I commit suicide I'll go to hell. I'm not up for it."

Using his logic, I try to move him away from the edge. "Joe, can you still get into heaven if you commit suicide slowly?"

"Hell yeah!"

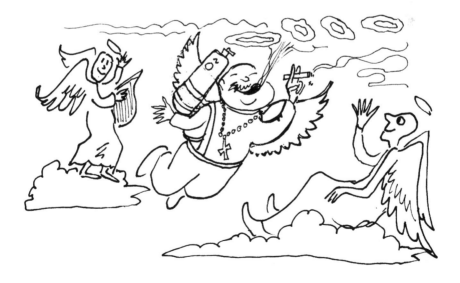

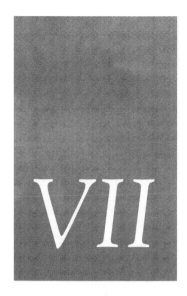

# On Love

Medicine is my beloved.
And that probably explains why I'm divorced
and living happily ever after.

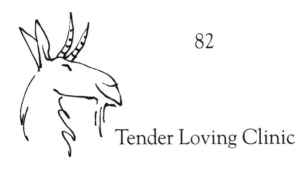

82

## Tender Loving Clinic

At thirty, I quit my first real job to open a clinic in my house for a year. I call it "Tender Loving Clinic." At TLC, I provide care to the uninsured—without time limits, corporate constraints, or other rules that don't serve people.

At my previous job, I had to see twenty-eight patients per day. One day—when another physician was out sick—I had to see forty-five patients!

There was no time to care, no time to properly diagnose or treat most patients. I questioned whether I was doing more harm than good.

To provide health care, I need time to care. So, at my house, every patient gets a sixty-minute appointment. TLC is my first experiment in designing a clinic, and I learn some important lessons.

Most people love longer visits, but not everyone. Some patients don't want tenderness, love, or care. They want antibiotics, narcotics, medical marijuana, or a note to get out of work.

Compared to women, men prefer shorter visits and less talking. They like to get in and out. Slam, bam, thank you Doc! Spending an hour with a man discussing his diet and exercise, his family and job, his joy and passion, and I'm in dangerous territory. Some men look at me funny, as if they think I'm flirting with them.

Apparently not everyone goes to the doctor for TLC. But it sure beats a TCE (Total Colon Examination) or a TWE (Tap Water Enema)!

# 83

# Love Is Medicine

It's Valentine's Day 1997, and I'm newly in love. I'm pretty much on my own for the night. I'm on call at my first job, while my Valentine—a wedding pianist—celebrates the nuptial bliss of a young newlywed couple in a penthouse restaurant just a few blocks away.

At Sacred Heart Hospital, I'm admitting a colleague's patient—an elderly man who is dying of heart disease. On oxygen, gasping for life, he exchanges no words. His wife—unable to bear the pain of watching him die—leaves the room. So it's just the two of us this Valentine's Eve. A blind date. No champagne. No candlelit dinner. I could leave too, but it doesn't seem right to let this guy die alone on this romantic day. So I sit with him, hold his hand, and cry.

A cardiologist looks in. Startled by my emotion, he says, "You must be a new doctor," then disappears down the hall.

Maybe old doctors don't cry, but I don't want to close my heart to the wounded.

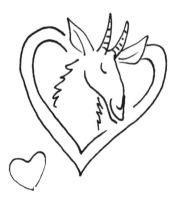

# 84

## Better Than Viagra—Part One

One of my sweetest patients is Johnny, an upbeat, fast-talking fellow in his mid-fifties. Johnny is disabled due to advanced arthritis that limits his mobility. Today, he returns for some advice. He says that he wants to stay active by volunteering and that he's ready for the companionship of a good woman.

His blood pressure has been creeping up over the last year, so I write two prescriptions. The first is a medication to lower his mildly elevated blood pressure. The second prescription reads: "Johnny is a great guy. He needs a wonderful woman in his life. I highly recommend him." As I'm reviewing his instructions, he leaps up from his chair to hug me.

Maybe I'm old-fashioned—I still handwrite prescriptions because what most patients really need can never be prescribed electronically.

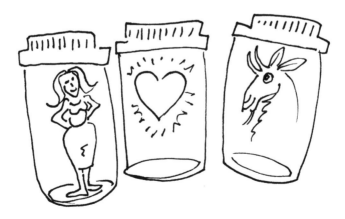

# 85

# Better Than Viagra—Part Two

One month later, Johnny returns for a blood pressure check.

"So, did you find a woman?" I ask.

Beaming, he replies, "I've been meaning to tell you what happened." He pulls out his neatly folded girlfriend-prescription stashed in his wallet and assures me that he will always be ready.

"No woman? So what happened?" I ask.

"I went to Walmart to turn in my blood pressure prescription. But when the pharmacist called me over to review the side effects, he mentioned my erections might not last as long! Well, I told him that won't work with my other prescription. So he asked to see my other prescription. After I handed it to him, he turned beet red—like Santa in a white lab coat! When the pharmacist finally looked up, he said, 'If that happens just skip a few days.'"

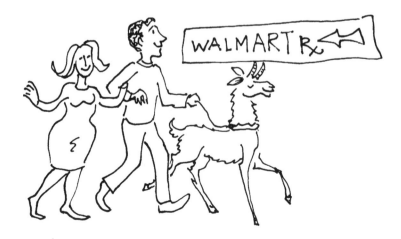

# 86

# Pap Prayer

Joy is a vibrant twenty-six-year-old woman who comes in for a physical. On her exam, she shows me a worrisome mole on her left shoulder. I recommend she return for removal. After the excision, I call her back to my office for results.

"You have a melanoma. We got it just in time, but I'm sending you to a dermatologist who will perform a wider excision—just to be safe. You should be fine."

She's concerned, but relieved. "What should I do?"

"We don't know the exact cause of melanoma. It's not like other skin cancers. You can get melanoma in areas of the body that are not exposed to the sun. A friend of mine [the illustrator of this book] developed melanoma inside her vagina—on her cervix!"

"So what do I do?" she begs.

"Keep your immune system strong. Avoid sunburns and carcinogens. Eat healthy. We'll do skin checks every year." As Joy's physician and friend, I'm also relieved. Melanoma can be fatal and metastasizes quickly. Had she waited a year, she could be dead.

Joy returns for her annual exams. It's been four years since her melanoma removal.

I call her with results the following week. "Your Pap smear looks great, but your test for human papillomavirus (HPV) reveals a high-risk strain that can predispose you to cervical cancer."

"What should I do, Pamela?"

"Don't worry. Though ninety-nine percent of cervical cancers are caused by HPV, most HPV infections resolve spontaneously. And most sexually active adults have had HPV. It's the most common sexually transmitted infection in the world."

"Weird. A sexual infection can cause cancer?" she asks.

"Yes. HPV-induced cancers can occur in the vagina, vulva, anus, and penis. It's also linked to cancers of the tongue, tonsils, and throat!"

"So what can I do to prevent getting cancer from the HPV infection?"

"There is an HPV vaccine that is approved for males and females age nine to twenty-six and is best given before any sexual activity. Since you've already been exposed, keep your immune system strong. Avoid smoking, alcohol, and carcinogens. Eat healthy. Be monogamous. The fewer partners the better! Come back next year and we'll do your Pap and HPV test again. Your body could clear the infection on its own."

"Is there anything else I can do?"

"Are you religious?"

"I have a spiritual practice," Joy says. "One of the things I do is meditate. Sometimes at an altar, such as my love altar."

"After your meditation, I'd like you to do a prayer to clear this virus from your body."

"Great. That's a wonderful idea."

A year later, Joy is back for her physical, repeat Pap, and HPV test.

"How are things going?"

"Oh, I'm in love! We are living together and things are great!"

"Awesome, Joy!"

As I perform her exam, I share the latest breakthroughs in Pap smear technology. "Joy, when I first trained, we had to twirl a small wooden spatula around the cervix and smear cervical cells and mucus onto a glass slide. Then we had to spray it right away with lots of hairspray!"

"Yuck!" she says.

"It was disgusting. I spent years coughing up hairspray fumes after Pap smears."

"But why hairspray?" Joy asks.

"It's a fixative for the cells. But some samples were still not adequate for analysis at the lab. So we'd have to call patients back for another smear and spray."

"Oh, that sounds awful," Joy says as I'm doing her Pap.

"Now we use a liquid Pap test. We rotate this little wiggly broom around the cervix and then swish it in this container of preservative solution. The lab can retrieve as many samples as they need from the liquid. They can do your Pap and HPV test, plus test for gonorrhea, chlamydia, herpes, cystic fibrosis—all from this tiny jar!"

"Amazing!" Joy exclaims.

"And no hairspray!" I add.

As Joy gets dressed, I label her specimen, drop it into a biohazard bag, and hand it to her.

"Here's your Pap. Take it home. Drop it off at the lab down the street in the next thirty days. You don't need to refrigerate it. Place your Pap on your prayer altar. You and your partner can do a special prayer together every night to release the HPV from your body."

"We'll do it, Pamela!" she says.

One month later I call Joy. "Did you do your Pap prayer?"

"Yes. We did it every evening and it brought us closer together. I really appreciated that we were able to connect spiritually."

"Great. You've got a normal Pap smear and no HPV!"

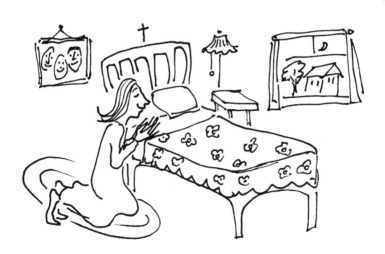

**"I pray for Mommy and Daddy, Aunt Flo, and my Pap smear."**

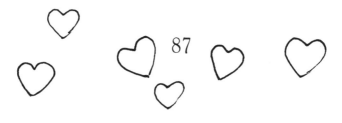

## 87

## I Love You!

Jill is a long-time patient. At the end of appointments she always says, "I love you!" Sometimes I whisper, other times I scream down the hall, "I love you too!"

I know I'm not supposed to tell patients I love them. But they tell me all the time. So if I'm feelin' it, I'm gonna say it.

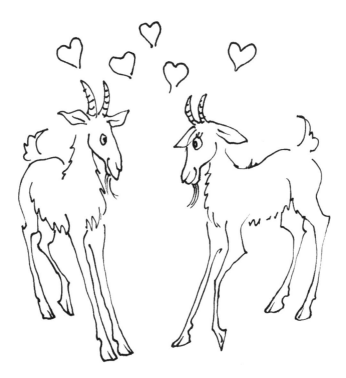

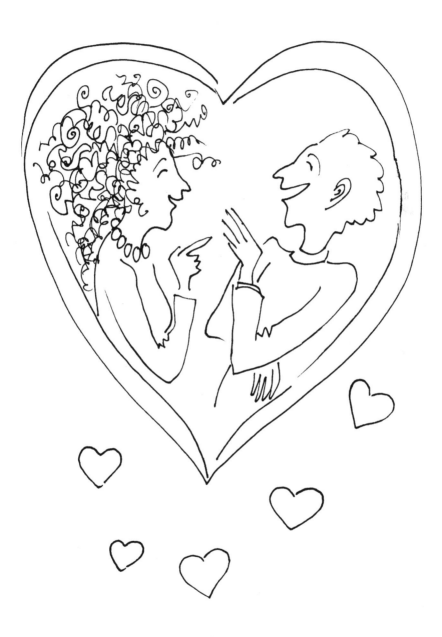

# 88

# Free Hugs

At the end of appointments many patients ask, "Can I get a hug?"

I always oblige. Afterward I pass along a "hug coupon" that can be used later. It's good for one free hug, redeemable from any consenting human being.

Many people don't know how to hug. That included me—till recently, when a patient taught me the proper way to give and receive a hug.

"Always reach out with the left arm," she explained, "so that both people are hugging heart-to-heart." She added, "If you are giving a hug, keep giving until the other person wants to let go."

Since I'm right-hand dominant, I've spent my entire life reaching out with my right (wrong) arm. I'm also guilty of ending hugs prematurely.

Doctors are perfectionists. We hate doing things the wrong way.

Hugging should be formally taught and tested in medical school. Students should feel comfortable in their ability to give and receive hugs before they begin caring for patients on clinical rotations.

When physicians can freely and spontaneously express affection with patients, we will be one step closer to providing comprehensive health care in America.

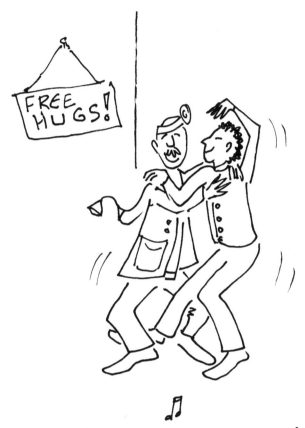

Ya put yer right arm in,
Ya put yer left arm out,
Ya put yer chest close in,
And ya smile without a pout.
Ya do the huggy-wuggy,
And ya twirl yerselves around.
That's what it's all about.

89

# Patient Appreciation Day

On random Fridays, clients are showered with extra affection to celebrate "Patient Appreciation Day." I surprise the unsuspecting visitors with dark-chocolate hearts and Mylar smiley-faced balloons as they enter the office. This is in addition to the gifts many receive for meeting their health goals. Sitting on the couch next to her balloon, treats piled high in her lap, a woman bursts out, "This is like going to Grandma's!"

Kids and adults alike enjoy the unexpected attention and gifts. It's especially exciting to surprise new patients, the ones who choose me at random from a preferred provider list given to them by their health insurance company. After receiving a door prize and an initial hour-long appointment, one woman exclaims, "I feel like I hit the lottery!"

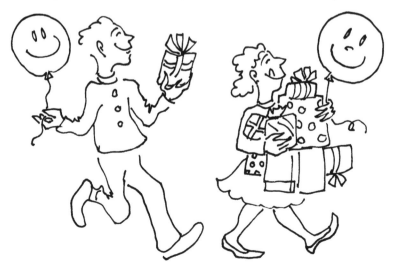

# 90

# The Raw Truth

I often wonder: Why am I a doctor?

The truth is, I want to live in the real world, a world without pretense, a world where people can't hide behind money or status.

Illness uncovers our authenticity. Doctoring satiates my need to be witnessed and to witness the raw, uncensored human experience. I crave intensity.

Like an emotional bungee jumper, I live to inhale the last words of a dying man, to hear the first cry of a newborn baby, to feel the slippery soft skin in my hands, to cut the cord and watch a drop of blood fall on my shoe, to wipe a new mother's tears, to introduce a father to his son, to hold a daughter's hand as she kisses her father good-bye one last time.

I am a doctor because I refuse to be numb. I want to live on the precipice of the underworld, the afterworld, to look into patients' eyes, to free-fall into an abyss of love, despair, death and then wake up tomorrow and do it all again.

Maybe doctoring fills a hole, a void. I doctor for connection, to be needed—to be loved.

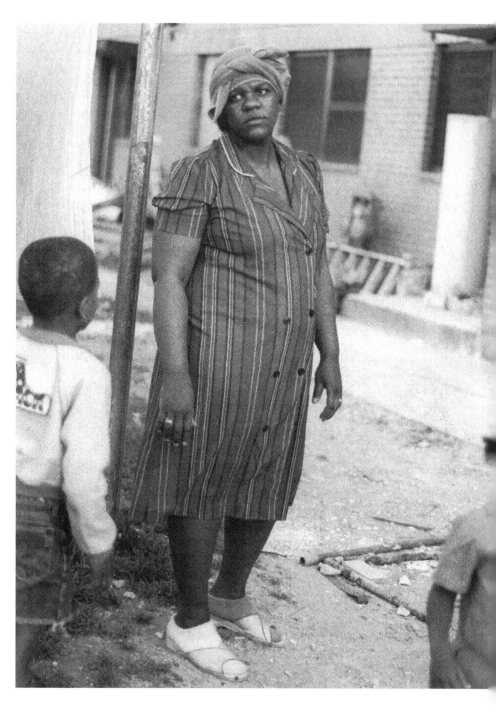

I took this picture of Albertha for my high school photography class.

# 91

# My Secret Godmother

Today, a reporter flies in from New Jersey to write a story on our community clinic. He audio records an afternoon of patients. At the end of each appointment he asks, "Why come to this clinic?"

"Coming to see Pamela is like visiting an angel," one woman says.

I'm humbled by my patients' love and admiration. For some patients, maybe a doctor is an answer to a prayer, an angel, or a saint.

I know a saint. My saint is from South Dallas. Her name is Albertha. Back in high school, I'm sixteen and dating her oldest son. He brings me home to the projects to meet his mom. Albertha is thirty years old with six kids, three jobs, and an unemployed husband. And she takes me under her wing.

Albertha is big and dark and strong, and she isn't afraid of me. Unlike other people, she never thinks I'm too intense, too emotional, or too idealistic. I'm never too much for her.

Albertha embodies the power of love. And her love is *for real*. When she says "I love you," I feel it in a place in my body that has never been touched.

Her life is hard, but I make her laugh. I follow her around the kitchen and to church with my tape recorder. I love her singing and her voice. I love her accent, how she says words, and how she puts sentences together. And I love her wild laughter. I keep telling her all the things I love about her, and that just makes her laugh more.

We exchange letters while I'm in college and medical school. She writes that—with God's help—I can be anything I want to be and that I can do anything I want to do. She always signs her envelopes: "You are loved." And I believe her.

When things get tough in school, I blast Albertha singing her gospel.

"We love your music," I tell Albertha.

She laughs, "Oh, Lord! You mean way over there in Boston they hearing my music?"

"Yep, you're popular in Boston."

"Oh, my God!" she laughs.

"It is so good! I just love it! My roommate can't stop listening to it!"

"I guess she can't help but listen to it if you gonna play it!"

"We just love your song!"

"What was I singing? Lord, have mercy!"

"That song 'I Have One More River to Cross.' I just love it!" It's an old Negro spiritual titled "Jordan River" in which Albertha sings of her death and reuniting with Jesus.

Years later, Albertha is dying of breast cancer at forty-nine. In her absence, I promise to look after her kids and grandkids.

Six years after her death, I get a call from her second-oldest son, Tonio. He tells me that Jordan—Albertha's oldest grandson—is in a foster home near Houston. "If my mama was alive," he says, "she'd never let Jordan be in foster care."

Fulfilling my promise, I phone Child Protective Services and say, "I'll take him."

"Who are you?" they ask.

"Umm . . . his paternal grandmother kind of adopted me when I was sixteen. I'm like his long-lost white aunt in Oregon."

They seem confused. I need a way to convince them that we are related.

Next week, I attend a family reunion in Texas with most of Albertha's family. Afterward, Tonio takes me to his apartment. He opens the hall closet and hands me a cardboard box. "This is everything my mama had on her nightstand when she died: her address book, her letters, and diary. I want you to have it 'cause you was closest to her."

I open the box and immediately smell her perfume. Then I pick up a small address book. I read it like a novel. At the end I find a list of my addresses. Printed above my name is: GODDAUGHTER.

I discover Albertha is my godmother!

I call Jordan's caseworker to inform her that "Jordan's paternal grand-mother is my godmother, so that makes me his fairy godmother aunt."

The state of Texas releases Jordan to my care. He's sixteen when he arrives and he stays for sixteen months. It's my honor to pass on to him the love that Albertha so freely shared with me when *I* was sixteen.

Albertha's love outlasts her lifetime. It flows through me every day to everyone I touch. Real love can't be contained. It must be passed on, released. Love must flow freely and fearlessly.

I'm not scared to love my patients. And my patients can choose to love me. If my patients want me to be their angel, saint, or secret godmother, who am I to resist?

Maybe that's why reporters keep coming to my office.

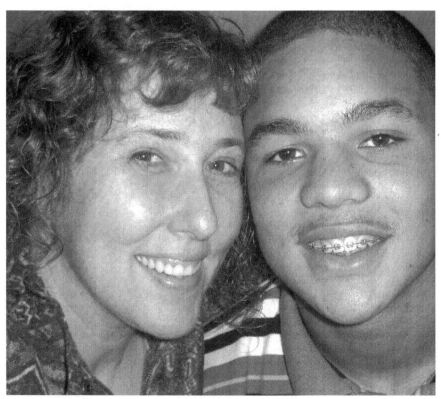

**Me and Jordan**

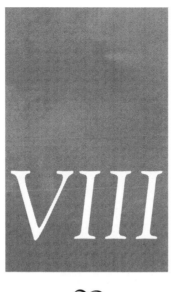

# VIII

## On Death

*When I die I want to reunite with my patients*
*so I can find out if they finally quit smoking.*

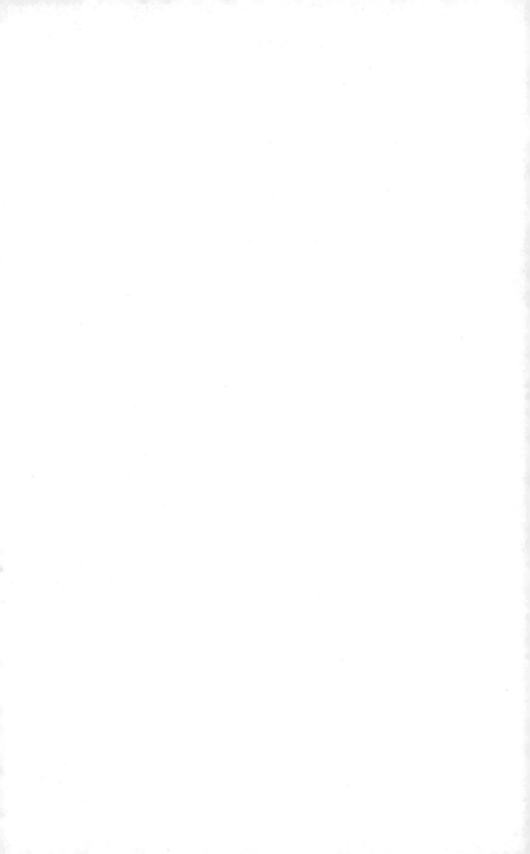

# 92

# Soul Sisters—Part One

Lily is a twenty-two-year-old Apache woman, with flyaway black hair and curious, playful eyes—with a sparkle of deviance. That's what attracts me to her. We meet at her hospital bed. I'm her new intern on the medical team.

Lily is no fan of the white man's world, but she trades her sweat lodge for a university hospital, her tribal shaman for a transplant surgeon.

Her lungs are failing; we are her only lifeline. She needs a lung transplant to survive.

Lily has idiopathic bronchiectasis: an irreversible destruction of her airways causing them to become widened and scarred. We have no idea why she developed this. Her condition may have been caused by infections that injured her lungs as a child. Now Lily's airways are losing the ability to clear mucus, dust, and bacteria—leading to additional infections and further destruction.

I'm a new doctor, just a few years older than Lily. I'm eager to discover how I may serve her, though I'm not exactly sure what to do. But I'm here. I'm energetic. And I'm ready.

I'll try to follow the lead of my superiors.

# 93

# Soul Sisters—Part Two

Lily is in and out of the hospital. But today, in clinic, we're celebrating. Lily has been accepted for a lung transplant! Now she wears a beeper to alert her at a moment's notice of an available donor. Weekly, she attends a transplant clinic. She pulls out a group photo. It's Lily with all her new friends awaiting lungs. The boy next to Lily has an X over his face and so does the woman behind her.

"So did those two get their lungs?" I ask.

"Nope," Lily says. "They died. I cross people off as they die."

To prepare for her new lungs, Lily is on an intensive medication regimen. But I discover she is not taking her medication. She doesn't want to. Like a wild horse, she wants to live but does not want to submit.

Today, I plead, "You're taking your inhalers four times per day, right?"

"Not really. Well, when I remember. Do I have to?"

"Lily! You have to take your treatments so your body will be in the best shape for surgery."

The next week, Lily is in the hospital with pneumonia. I sit with the transplant team as we discuss her case. I share that Lily is not compliant with her medications. We know that if she won't take her medications, her body will reject her new lungs—lungs that could go to another patient in need.

As a result, Lily is declared ineligible for a transplant. I deliver her death sentence. Hysterical, she throws her dinner tray at the nurse. She sobs uncontrollably, her body violently shaking in bed.

I never leave her side.

The transplant team signs off on Lily's case. "We have nothing left to offer her." I look to my superiors for guidance. "There's nothing much we can do now," they say.

So I sneak my dog, Happy, into Lily's room at night for impromptu excursions. As the miniature collie lunges forward, I grip his leash with one hand and pull Lily out of bed with the other, her portable oxygen tank rolling behind.

We exit the hospital and disappear into a blanket of grass and gaze at the stars. On these midnight escapades, Lily feels good, but she also shares the grief of never giving birth or meeting her soul mate. I hint at adventures yet to come while making lists of things Lily can still enjoy.

One night while we are giggling, I grab Lily's hand and lead her into the parking garage to show her my pickup truck. I just painted it with Dr. Seuss characters and the phrase: FEELS GOOD! I whisk her away for a ride around town, windows down, our hair flying in the wind.

Before we head back to the hospital, I say, "How 'bout ice cream?"

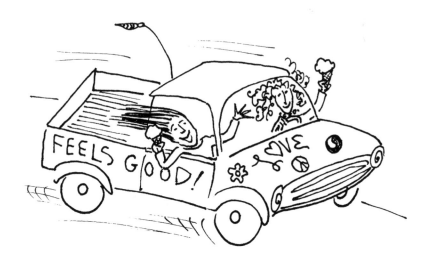

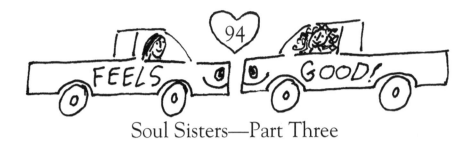

## Soul Sisters—Part Three

Lily returns to the clinic a few days later for our hospital follow-up appointment. When I open the exam room door, I'm captivated by her mischievous grin. She removes her oxygen, grabs my hand, then pulls me down the hall.

Breathless, in her raspy voice, she boasts, "Pamela, I did what you told me to do."

"Oh no. What did I tell you to do?"

Lily leads me to a Nissan pickup truck parked next to mine. Both pickups are covered with hand-painted cartoons and the words: "FEELS GOOD!" Wow. Lily has the same exact pickup truck! And she painted it to match mine! The only difference is her pickup has Disney characters and mine has Dr. Seuss.

*Nissan*—of Hebrew origin—means miracle. And I marvel at the sight: Two Nissan pickups—white with maroon interiors—side by side, hers and mine. I never told her to do it, but if Lily and I were pickups, this is what we'd look like.

White-coated colleagues assemble in the parking lot to examine the matching physician-patient pickups, and they file back into the clinic without a word.

Months later, at her home, surrounded by family, I sit with Lily—her cold body wrapped in a plush Mickey Mouse blanket—then I kiss her goodbye and sign her body over to the morgue.

But Lily never leaves my side.

Her Nissan, now driven by her sister, follows me all around town.

When I think of Lily, I look out the window and see Mickey, reminding me that Lily feels good.

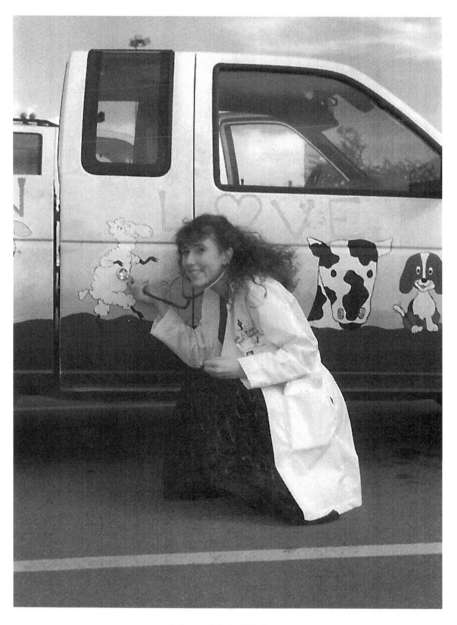

**Me and My Pickup**

# 95

# Buddha Babies

Raised in a morgue, I spent my childhood accompanying my dad to the hospital mortuary where I followed him around at work. I peeked in on autopsies and examined body parts, but I was most intrigued by the babies. They looked like Buddhas. From largest to smallest, they sat cross-legged along the shelf. Floating in jars, they leaned toward me and stared straight through me. And they never blinked. They seemed to know something I didn't. But who were they? And why were *they* trapped in jars? And how come I wasn't inside a jar, too?

My dad's inner-city miscarriage collection still intrigues me. All Philadelphia natives, they were probably Irish Catholic, Puerto Rican, and mostly African American. But none were black, or brown, or white. All blue babies. All race-neutral. Chromosomal defects were the likely cause of demise. Maybe their tender souls weren't ready for a rough, urban life.

When Dad retired, he offered me his miscarriage collection. I was honored to be asked to watch over their little bodies rather than have them incinerated as medical waste. But I could not see stuffing all the jars into my carry-on bag and holding up the line at the airport while trying to explain myself. So I kept only one. I made it through airport security with that tiny person in my pocket—a six-week-old calcified embryo about the size of a pebble.

Sometimes when I lose sight of the big picture, I hold that tiny person in my hand and I see the whole world.

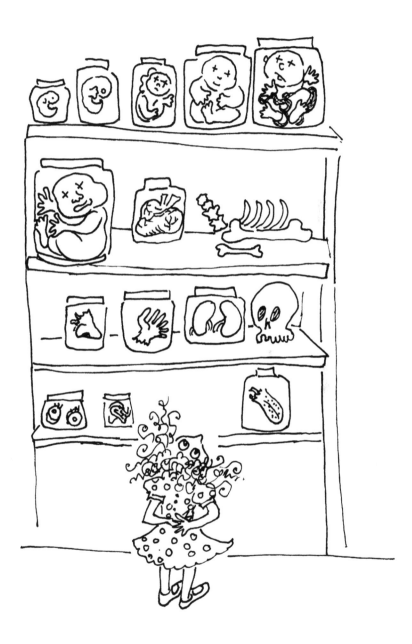

# 96

# Hitchhiking for Health Care

Harry is a quirky fifty-eight-year-old recluse, balding with clumps of wavy brown hair held back in a rubber band. He wears leather boots, loose cotton pants, and a purple sweatshirt that smells of sweet incense and cedar.

Harry lives in a small cabin, and he caretakes a wildlife sanctuary surrounded by a national forest. It's a simple life with no running water or electricity. He has no phone or car. But—surprisingly—he does have health insurance. Covered by his employer, he can choose any doctor he likes. His ex-girlfriend recommended me three years ago; he's been hitching rides to my office ever since.

The nearest town is ten miles down a winding road. There's nothing much there, certainly no doctors. But continuing fifty miles west on Highway 22 is the capital: Salem, Oregon. There's every kind of doctor a man could want in Salem, but not for Harry. He's in it for the long haul with me. It's another hour and a half down Interstate 5 before he's dropped off at my office. It's a three-hour drive one-way, on a good day. Today it's snowing. Chains or snow tires are required for mountain roads and the highway is coated with ice.

But nothing stops Harry.

Patient loyalty is endearing. Some patients refuse to see any other doctor—they'd rather wait it out or die at home. It's an intense devotion that I've never experienced in my personal life. And how can I ever reciprocate? Maybe I shouldn't even try.

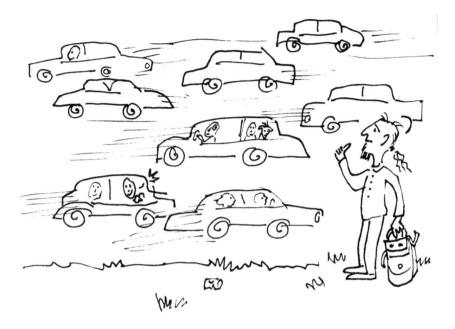

There's a backstory behind every disease: Harry develops a large, ulcerated boil on his cheek. Soon his back is covered in lumps, some so large it's painful to sleep. He agrees to surgery. With a stainless-steel scalpel, I excise a fibrous yellow mass behind his right shoulder. I sew him up, offer a hug, a kiss on the forehead, and provide a slip for a chest X-ray and schedule an appointment to return next week.

I don't share bad news by phone. At his next appointment, I lean forward and look into Harry's eyes. "The tests show a ten-centimeter cancer in the left upper lung that has metastasized to the back and face."

His voice cracks, eyes tear. A gulp. Silence.

I wonder about wounds. As I stare at his chest X-ray, I wonder how a cancer can grow so large as to completely obscure one's heart.

Harry wants to fight. I've watched these fights before. I don't believe in fighting though. I believe death can be graceful, beautiful.

Harry moves to town for chemo. He gets a cell phone and finds a two-story house for reduced rent in exchange for pet-sitting several cats. I treat him to breakfast at a downtown café, then we walk to the corner bookstore. He tells me his place smells of cigarettes and wonders whether that will adversely impact his recovery. After twenty-four years of smoking, he quit at forty-two. The smell gets to him now.

Weeks pass. I'm sitting with Harry on the couch where he sleeps blanketed in cats. He feels "beat up" from chemo. Now the cancer center won't see him without a credit card. Insurance stopped paying me too, but he doesn't need to know.

"How's the pain?" I ask.

"It's increasing, but I'm opening up in a new way. It's a powerful process." Harry is so frail he must be carried upstairs to the bathroom, but he insists he's fine. He tells me that he's looking for another rental. "I'll be moving soon to a new place—a place without cats, without smoke, without a stairwell."

"I know that place, Harry. Let's go home."

He nods.

Surrounded by friends, he dies the next afternoon in his cabin, his ashes now food for the forest he so loved.

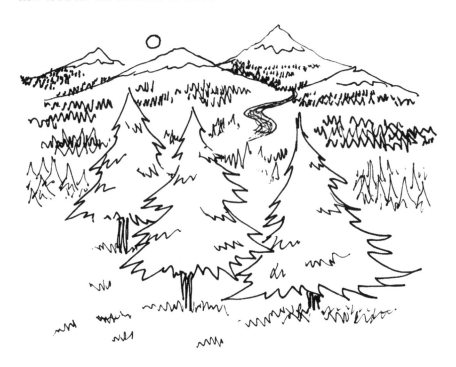

# 97

# Dying Healthy

As I get older, I'm less interested in forcing people into standard algorithms and more intrigued to discover what people really want from me. Now I ask patients directly, "What are your health goals?"

One man says: "Run a marathon and die in my sleep when I'm 120."

Another woman's goal: "I want to die healthy."

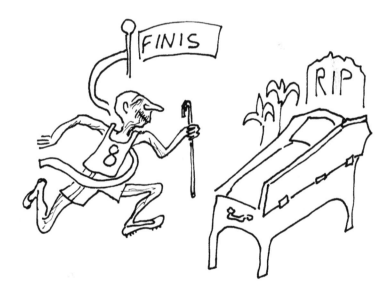

# 98

# Death Row

Texas leads the nation in executions.

As a medical student at University of Texas Medical Branch at Galveston, I provided health care for Texas prison system inmates, many on death row. In fact, the prison hospital is conveniently attached to the main university hospital.

Anytime, day or night, with a flash of my school ID, the guards press a button and I'm in. The massive door opens ahead of me. Then a series of steel gates unlocks one by one as I pass rows of caged men.

Death-row health care is an oxymoron. How do I reconcile "first do no harm" with the death penalty? How do I care for someone soon to be killed? I'm only twenty-three years old. Medical school doesn't prepare me for this. They just send me in here.

I believe all patients deserve the same kindness and respect. But it's not the same here. I'm in a place where "How are you?" is a loaded question, a place where men find Jesus and prepare their last statements before lethal injections.

I enter a cell. Sitting in front of me is a white man in his fifties recovering from a hernia repair. As I take his blood pressure and listen to his heart, I wonder how many people he may have shot or stabbed.

"Blood pressure is normal. Your heart's good."

"Thanks, Doc."

He disrobes and I examine his groin incision and his genitals. And I wonder how many women he may have raped or dismembered.

"You're healing just fine. No signs of infection."

I flip through his chart to see how I may best serve him. I notice his cholesterol is high.

"When was your last complete physical exam?"

"They check me pretty regular," he says.

Here's where it gets really confusing. He's due for a colonoscopy, but do we do colonoscopies before executions? And I want to discuss his cholesterol, but first I need to know one thing: can death-row inmates get heart-healthy meals?

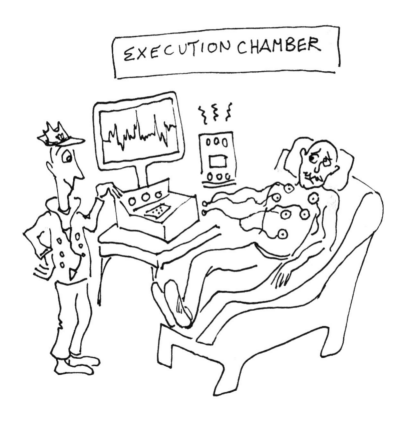

**"We're just hooking you up to the EKG to be sure you've got a good, strong heart."**

# 99

## Robert-Assisted Suicide—Part One

Robert is a bad patient with a bad disease. He hasn't always followed my advice. In fact, I've almost fired him twice, but he keeps coming back.

"Robert, if you don't want to follow my advice, why do you want me to be your doctor?"

"To give me the good stuff in case I'm gonna croak," he says.

I've taken care of Robert for six years now. Robert has had a rough life. He grew up on the South Side of Chicago, the only white kid in the 'hood. He got beat up a lot. Now Robert is sixty with kidney failure and horrible gout. His joints are so deformed he can't bend them. Some open up and weep. His brother just died of the same thing last month.

Robert lives in the woods with his wife, Linda. They tell me it was love at first sight. They met and were engaged twenty-four hours later. They've been married twenty-five years. They live off the land. Raise sheep and goats. She knits and sells felted crafts. He's a carpenter. Now he can't work. They pay twenty to forty dollars per visit when they have it.

When Robert first came to me, his blood pressure was so high I thought he'd have a stroke. I put him on medication. He didn't always take it. Three months later he had a stroke. He couldn't move his right arm or leg much and had to go hopping to the outhouse. He didn't seek treatment for days because his psychic medicine friend said he didn't need to go to the hospital. His psychic friend may know something I don't. But I know Robert. He didn't want to run up a big bill and leave his wife homeless. He learned to walk again on his own. He hobbles now.

I asked Robert to see a kidney specialist. The initial visit was $450. He couldn't afford it, but we finally got him in as a charity case. The kidney doctor gave him "a few more years to live" and started him on a drug that made his skin peel off and most of his hair fall out. So he quit the drug.

Robert is in a lot of pain. We've tried a lot of drugs. Medical marijuana and vodka work best. Linda is so upset that she cries through Robert's appointments. After screaming at me once and not following her own medical plan, I fired Linda as a patient. But we get along great now. Today they're back in the office.

"I feel depressed," Robert says, "though not suicidal. It's the pain that's getting me, Doc. When things get real bad, I plan to stop eating. How 'bout the suicide pill?"

I pause.

Finally I respond, "Here's a prescription for some morphine tablets. Let's see if this will work for your pain. I've never had anyone request physician-assisted suicide, but it is legal in Oregon."

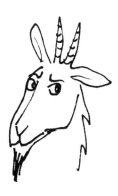

# 100

# Robert-Assisted Suicide—Part Two

Linda calls. "Robert has the heebie-jeebies and was all over the bed last night like a jumping bean, majorly twitchy."

She puts Robert on the phone.

"What's going on, Robert?"

"I feel like I'm being duct-taped down. Can't breathe. It starts with a sensation of warmth and then I gotta take off my clothes 'cause I feel restricted. I feel like I'm dying. I got a loaded pistol by my bed. If it gets bad I'm gonna shoot myself in the head, Doc."

"No," I beg. "Please don't do it." I imagine Linda cleaning blood and brains off the couch as her last memory of Robert. "Hey, you don't have to suffer. I researched what we need to do to meet the requirements of the Death with Dignity Act. You just need to make two oral requests fifteen days apart. You already made your first request last month. So now we just complete some forms. It's simple. We'll need another doctor to cosign. I'll track down your kidney doc to see if he'll do it. For now, let's try a fast-acting tranquilizer for panic and a heavy-duty pain patch to keep you comfortable."

A week later, I drive about an hour down a country road to their house.

Linda greets me at the gravel driveway and leads me into their rustic wooden yurt.

On the way in, Linda explains, "At your request, I spoke with hospice today, but we're not interested. Robert has six pain patches on and this seems to help him sleep."

Robert is on the couch. "Hey, Robert. How ya doing?"

"I haven't left home in a month, Doc. Been on the couch mostly 'cause of dizziness, weakness, and pain. Not eating or peeing much. Having bowel movements every three days. I'm on Vodka and the patches."

Robert is ninety pounds. He speaks softly, but coherently, and is of sound mind to sign the forms. His family concurs with the decision. A witness is here to confirm. Now I'm making mental notes about what I need to do next. I need a second physician to sign his form. If I can't get his kidney doc, I'll start begging my physician friends in town.

Then I explain, "Once I get this form signed by a second doctor, I'll write a prescription for ten grams of Seconal that you can administer yourself within the next forty-eight hours. Okay, Robert? Don't shoot yourself. Linda, call the pharmacies to make sure it's in stock. I'll be in touch."

I phone his kidney doctor. He is willing to sign.

I alert Linda. "I got the second doctor. I'm getting the forms signed. So we should be set for tomorrow. Did you find the Seconal?"

"I found it at only one pharmacy," Linda says. "It's $637!"

"What? That's insane!" I exclaim. "It's generic. These pills should cost five cents. This stuff has been on the market for, like, fifty years. Dad had hundreds of tablets in a huge stock bottle stored in our basement when I was a kid."

"Hey," Linda replies, "with my handy-dandy Oregon Prescription Drug Program discount card you told me to get, they plan to charge me only $550."

The next day, the kidney doctor calls to say he has second thoughts.

"Why?" I ask.

"As I remember, this guy is a psychiatric case," he says.

"What?"

"This guy has a psych history."

"Robert's a good guy," I explain. "He chooses to live off the grid in the woods with his wife. He is ninety pounds and on the couch dying. You know he has kidney failure. But if you don't feel comfortable, I'll find another doctor. Thanks anyway."

I call Linda. "We got problems. The kidney doctor backed out. I'm pissed, but I'm searching for another doctor to help us. Don't buy the drug yet. In the meantime, I want you to keep him comfortable with pain patches."

"Will do, Doc."

Two days later, I'm still not able to find another doctor willing to sign the Death with Dignity form. The next afternoon, Robert dies in his sleep.

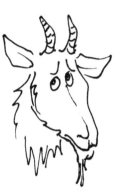

# 101

## Robert-Assisted Suicide—Part Three

It has been a year since Robert died. Linda moved to California to be near her kids. I follow her on Facebook.

I message her today: "Linda, I'm writing a book with 101 patient stories. I want to include Robert's story. Can you check in with him and make sure it's okay?"

"Hey, my dear," she replies. "Got a message from Robert. He showed up at the dentist's office. Hate typing. I'll call and leave the story on your voicemail."

The following day I receive this message:

> Hi, Doctor Pam. This is Linda with a story about Robert and the dentist. As an aside, I'll say that he's been hanging around, except for a little bit at Christmas. And I get communications from him on my right shoulder in varying degrees and volumes, depending on the nature of the issue.
>
> But at the dentist's office, I actually saw him. I had a couple of molars that were in need of removal. I put it off from last summer, but had to finally do it. It got a bit arduous at one point. They were holding open my jaw with a lot of pressure, trying to get some buried roots in there.
>
> Suddenly, Robert appeared right where the dentist's light is up there, between the faces of the assistant and the dentist. And he looked great, Doctor Wible! He was all smiling and his hair was thick and brown and long, and his

beard was black again. That was very cool.

He held out his hands. In the center of each palm was an indigo spot, and from each spot issued forth a kind of milky, square beam of golden light. He aimed them into my mouth where the doctor was working and, after a bit, he aimed one at the assistant and then he aimed them both at the dentist. And just then the dentist said, 'This is going very well!' It was so cool.

Oh, and Robert says he's fine with you including his story in the book. Hey, carry on the good work, my dear.

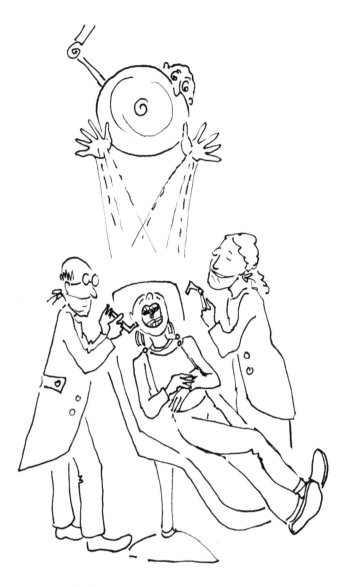

Robert returns as the Tooth Fairy.

# Imagine . . .

### Design . . . Draw . . . Dream . . . **Your Ideal Clinic** . . .

# Imagine . . .

Design . . . Draw . . . Dream . . . **Your Ideal Doctor** . . .

# Epilogue

# Live Your Dreams!

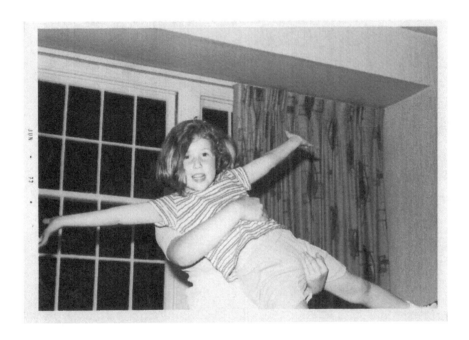

# Acknowledgments

Nothing is random. The convergence of many lives made this book possible.

I had been trying to write a book for five years. I attended writing conferences. I won awards on sample chapters. I had an agent, Diane Freed, whom I adored. Diane submitted my book proposal to the big publishers. I was so excited. But they weren't as excited about my book. So I revised. I rewrote. I struggled. My book became a burden. I lost interest and gave up.

Why? I had been writing the wrong book. At the wrong time. Synchronicity was not on my side.

Then one day, I parted with my agent and stopped listening to the advice of traditional publishers. And I started to hear my own voice and the voices of my patients who live inside me. And their voices were so loud that I couldn't sleep at night. All I wanted to do was write, and laugh, and love their stories. And I did.

I wrote this book in a little over a month. No burden. No struggle. Pure joy. And then, all the right people (and a pet goat) appeared. Just at the right time. Perfect synchronicity.

In the fall of 2004, I had dropped out of medicine and decided to return to waitressing. Then a bizarre set of circumstances led me to a self-care retreat. There, I met Kassy Daggett, the workshop leader. She performed some type of spiritual CPR on me. And she saved my career. Kassy became my therapist and friend. She is also my patient and the star of the Self-Papping chapter. To say we have a close relationship is an understatement. She is now co-leading workshops with me to help save my colleagues' careers and, of course, she just happens to be a graphic designer. Obviously, I chose her to design and format this book. Thank you, Kassy!

In 2008, I met Betsy Robinson in New York City while I was speaking with national media. She immediately understood me and became energized about community-designed health care. Betsy saw potential in me that I was unable to see in myself. She helped get my first national article published in *Spirituality & Health* and has remained my editor ever since. Thank you for believing in me, Betsy.

I met William Smith when he crashed my birthday party a few years ago. I usually run into William around eleven o'clock in the evening at the grocery store. Sometimes, after shopping, we sit outside on a bench immersed in late-night conversation until sunrise. I wanted a male perspective on my writing and William is a very thoughtful and sensitive man. He read, commented on, and edited my chapters twice weekly as I wrote them. We did not always agree and sometimes I offended him. I thank you, William, for your clarity and for hanging in there with me past midnight when I was stubborn, irritable, and exhausted.

Bo Adan popped into my life at the last possible moment before I completed my final manuscript. Thanks for the copious notes and meticulous editing, Bo. You definitely deserve a tip. And then Leigh Anne Jasheway appeared out of nowhere to assist with comic editing. She helped turn my amusing prose and cartoon captions into actual comedy.

Sydney Ashland is one amazing woman. She is my colleague, therapist, spiritual advisor, and friend. I met with Sydney weekly while writing this book. She read my chapters as I wrote them and offered incredible insight and direction. I can never thank you enough for everything you have done for me, Sydney.

Nearly 100 teenagers, medical students, and physicians reviewed the manuscript prior to publication. Thank you all for helping me turn a rough draft into a real book.

I'd like to give a special shout-out to the amazing citizens in my hometown. To those of you who attended the town hall meetings, I am forever thankful. You have made Eugene, Oregon, the epicenter of a national movement for ideal medical care. And most importantly, I thank my patients for allowing me to share your stories with the world. I love you all!

So many others provided inspiration, assistance, and feedback along the way. In particular I'm grateful for Francine Porter, Mariah Stevens, Sherri Brown, Trisha Maxfield, Spark Boemi, Michael Backus, Bodhi Goforth, Chris Flores, M.D., Jane Powers, Kathy Smyly Miller, Steve Harrison, Jack Canfield, Darren Hunt, Nancy Wood, Stella Verdouw, Arun Toké,

Luminara Serdar, Scott Gray, Jeya Aerenson, Sue Goldish, Tanja Petal, Amanda Everett, Steve Frankel, Gale Fiszman, Rachel Farkas, Indya Bull, Jeff Cochran, Brooke Morris, Chase Bain, Daphne Gabrieli, Heesang Byun, and for Jonathan Boone—come home from Afghanistan and make music, not war! We need a movie soundtrack for *Pet Goats & Pap Smears*, dude.

And, of course, I thank the pet goat! I spent months looking for a therapy goat for my office. Then I ended up meeting the perfect goat, Charity, through a soap-making class I attended with my mom.

I told Mom, "I'm writing a book. I don't have time to make soap!"

She begged me to go.

When I arrived at the soap-making class, I put in my earplugs and spent the entire time revising *Pet Goats & Pap Smears*—until I overheard women discussing goat's-milk soap. I removed my earplugs just as Aida Camalich Lough raised her hand to announce she had relocated here from Los Angeles with her mobile petting zoo—with fifteen therapy goats! Thank you, Aida, for bringing these beautiful goats into my life.

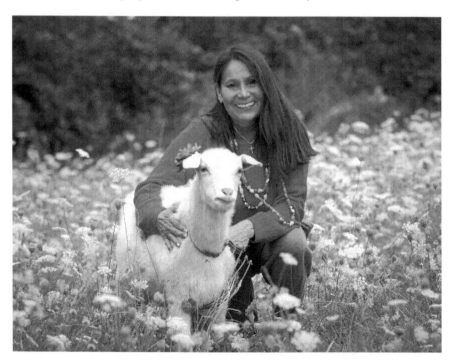

**Charity and Aida**

I thank my mother for being a medical pioneer in her own right:

> In 1965 my mother, Judith Wible, received her medical degree from the University of Texas Medical Branch at Galveston. Of 160 graduates, eight were female. The dean and fellow students reminded the 'girls' in the class that they were 'taking a man's seat' and they would never use their degrees. Even the anatomy professor refused to accept female anatomy and persisted in addressing women as men. Despite her protests, my mother remained 'Mr. Wible.' Women were excluded from urology—from palpating penises and prostates—while men dominated obstetrics and gynecology. Daily, the women were exposed to filthy jokes that demeaned female patients, and in the evenings they slept in cramped nursing quarters while the guys had fraternities complete with maids, cooks, parties, and last year's exams.
>
> ~ *Goddess Shift: Women Leading for a Change*, Elite Books, 2011

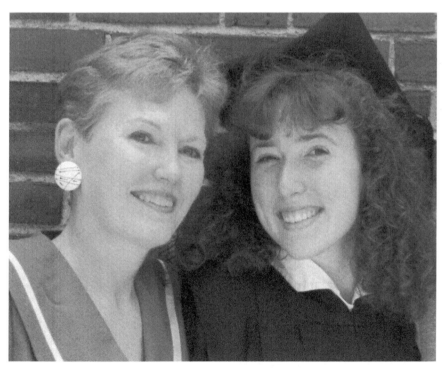

**Wellesley College Graduation. Thanks for everything, Mom!**

# ACKNOWLEDGMENTS

My dear friend, Kiki Metzler, was sitting in her backyard imagining her perfect illustration gig when I hired her to illustrate this book. Kiki is the perfect cartoonist for a book on Pap smear adventures. Why? She survived melanoma of the cervix. At the time of her diagnosis, there were only twelve reported cases in the world. Kiki, I am so fortunate to have you in my life. Stick around. I've got more books for you to illustrate.

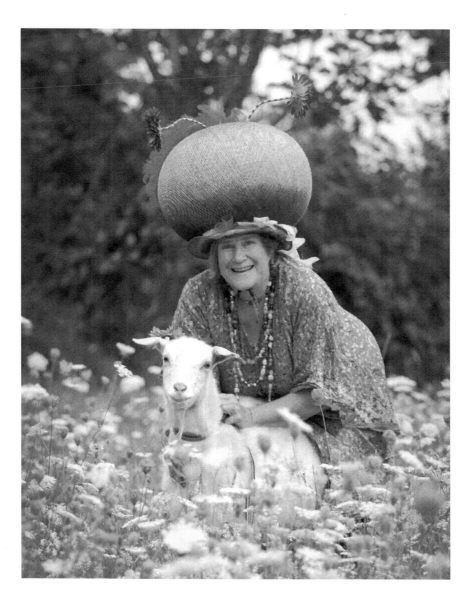

# Resources

## Want Ideal Medical Care?

Join the ideal medical care movement at www.idealmedicalcare.org. Explore the map of ideal clinics nationwide. Find one near you or start your own! Host a town hall meeting in your community and invite Dr. Wible.

## Share *Pet Goats & Pap Smears*

Go to www.petgoatsandpapsmears.com to buy the book for your friends and family. All book proceeds will be used to help communities create their own ideal clinics.

## Bulk Orders

Dr. Pamela Wible is available to speak at colleges, universities, and medical schools. It is her dream that all premedical and medical students will receive a copy of this book. For pricing on bulk orders or to schedule Dr. Wible for your next event, contact: www.petgoatsandpapsmears.com.

## Books Coauthored by Pamela Wible, M.D.

*Goddess Shift: Women Leading for a Change* (Elite Books, 2011)

*Optimism: Cultivating the Magic Quality that Can Extend Your Lifespan, Boost Your Energy, and Make You Happy Now* (Elite Books, 2012)

# Retreats

### *Live Your Dream: Revolutionize Your Practice*
Pamela Wible, M.D. & Kassy Daggett, L.M.T.

Take refuge with like-minded colleagues who realize healing health care begins within. . . . Reclaim your vision, then liberate yourself to practice medicine in alignment with your values—and the values of your community. Rest, replenish, and retreat with kindred spirits while mastering the business, leadership, and community organizing skills you never learned in school. This workshop is open to doctors, medical students, nurses, hospital CEOs, massage therapists—everyone in health care!
Contact: www.idealmedicalcare.org

CAUTION: If you are happy with health care in America, do not attend this workshop.


### *Self Care on the Path of Service*
Kassy Daggett, L.M.T. & Victor Rozek, certified coach

Once we are called to the path of service, it can be challenging to remain available for others when our own life events become overwhelming. This retreat offers an opportunity to do deep, personal work and clear feelings of sacrifice, fatigue, and burnout. Take time to actively breathe spirit back into your life and clear the way for being fully present with others. This workshop is designed for everyone in health care and anyone who walks the path of service.
Contact: www.vrkd.com

WARNING: This is the retreat that saved Dr. Wible's career.

*Pet Goats & Pap Smears*
Reading Group Guide

*This guide is offered to book clubs, schools, families, friends, and individuals who wish to deepen their understanding of topics presented in this book.*

# Discussion Questions

## I. Ideal Medical Care

1. What does ideal health care mean to you?

2. Describe your ideal clinic.

3. Would you like to create an ideal clinic for your neighborhood?

4. Describe your ideal doctor.

5. Would you share this book with your doctor? Why? Why not?

6. Does health insurance equal health care?

7. Do you believe that national health care reform can deliver ideal medical care for all? If not, describe how this could be achieved.

8. What do you believe is the solution for our health care system? Who would implement the solution?

## II. General *Pet Goat & Pap Smears* Topics

1. What one new fact did you learn from the book, and why is it important to you?

2. Have you shared any stories from this book with friends or family members? Why? Why not?

3. What surprised you most?

4. Would you recommend this book to others? Why?

5. Would you recommend this book to teenagers? If not, why?

6. Do you believe children should be exposed to death at a young age? If your child expressed an interest in anatomy, would you allow him or her to view an autopsy? Why? Why not?

7. Should young children be permitted to accompany their parents to work? In what circumstances would this not be appropriate?

8. Do you think the illustrations enhance the stories? How so?

9. What was your reaction to the book cover?

10. Are the issues raised in the book controversial?

11. Share specific passages that struck you as most significant.

12. What was most amusing? Did you laugh out loud?

13. What was most profound? Why?

14. What part of the book did you find most intriguing? Why?

15. What was the most memorable part of this book for you? Why?

## III. Physicians & Medicine

1. What have you learned that may change the way you interact with your doctor?

2. What unique prescription would you like to receive from your doctor?

3. Did you realize that, in the past, most doctors were required to kill dogs as part of their training? What impact do you think such experiences have on physicians?

4. How do you feel about doctors maintaining a "professional distance" from patients?

5. Is it okay to hug your doctor?

6. Is it okay to speak to your doctor on a first-name basis?

7. Is it okay to tell your doctor that you love her/him?

8. Did you learn about any unusual illnesses from reading this book?

9. What treatments in this book did you find surprising?

10. What did you learn about Pap smears?

11. Did you learn anything new about sexually transmitted infections?

## IV. Money

1. In chapter 16, the Amish want a fair bill. What does *a fair bill* mean to you?

2. Do you believe self-pay patients should be given a discount?

3. Should patients who are religiously opposed to lawsuits be given discounts?

4. Do you believe that all Americans should buy health insurance?

5. Should people who are religiously or politically opposed to purchasing health insurance be forced to buy insurance? Why? Why not?

6. How do you feel about billing doctors for excessive waiting?

7. Would you ever give your doctor a tip for fabulous service?


## V. Politics

1. How do you feel about capital punishment and physician-assisted suicide?

2. What is your view on prostitution? Has your view changed since reading this book?

3. In chapter 51, what did you think about Melissa's job as a sex worker? Should she be permitted to work legally?

4. What is your view on medical marijuana? Has your view changed since reading this book?

5. How do you feel about incarcerating nonviolent drug offenders?

6. Does our culture support honest, open communication about sexuality? Why? Why not?

7. Are abstinence-only programs effective?

8. Do you support sex education in the schools? At what age is it appropriate to begin sex education?

## VI. Life Lessons

1. Is there a take-away lesson from this book that will change your life? What is it? Explain why this is important to you.

2. What other life lessons can be learned from this book?

3. Did you have any preconceived notions about doctors or about the health care system that have changed after reading these stories? Please explain and share the chapter that made you reconsider your position.

4. Do you believe anyone can be revolutionary just by being happy?

5. Did you learn anything new about intimate relationships?

6. Did you learn anything new about gender differences?

7. Did you learn anything new about interpersonal communication?

8. Do you remember your childhood dream?

9. Are you living your dream?

10. If you are not living your dream, what's stopping you?

Have *you* hugged
your doctor today?

Made in the USA
San Bernardino, CA
22 August 2015